Women's Cancers

Pathways to Living

Women's Cancers

Pathways to Living

J Richard Smith

Imperial College, UK &
New York University School of Medicine, USA

Giuseppe Del Priore

Cancer Treatment Centers of America &
Morehouse School of Medicine, USA

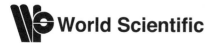 World Scientific

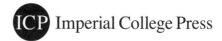 Imperial College Press

Published by

Imperial College Press
57 Shelton Street
Covent Garden
London WC2H 9HE

Distributed by

World Scientific Publishing Co. Pte. Ltd.
5 Toh Tuck Link, Singapore 596224
USA office: 27 Warren Street, Suite 401-402, Hackensack, NJ 07601
UK office: 57 Shelton Street, Covent Garden, London WC2H 9HE

Library of Congress Cataloging-in-Publication Data
Smith, J. Richard.
 Women's cancers : pathways to living / J Richard Smith, Imperial College, UK & New York
University, USA, Giuseppe Del Priore, Cancer Treatment Centers of America & Morehouse School
of Medicine, USA.
  pages cm
 Includes bibliographical references and index.
 ISBN 978-1-78326-729-3 (hardcover : alk. paper) -- ISBN 978-1-78326-730-9 (pbk. : alk. paper)
 1. Cancer in women--Popular works. I. Del Priore, Giuseppe. II. Title.
 RC281.W65S66 2015
 616.99'40082--dc23
                                                     2015021510

British Library Cataloguing-in-Publication Data
A catalogue record for this book is available from the British Library.

Typeset by Stallion Press
Email: enquiries@stallionpress.com

Printed by FuIsland Offset Printing (S) Pte Ltd Singapore

This book is dedicated to all those women who we, as a team, have had the privilege to look after and who have encouraged the use of the 4 cusp approach and, thus, this project.

"Above all, what matters is not to lose the joy of living for the fear of dying."

Maggie Keswick Jencks, Co-founder of Maggie's Cancer Caring Centres

By kind permission of Laura Lee CEO Maggie's

Acknowledgements

This book is an updated version of a previous book, *Women's Cancers: Pathways to Healing*. As such, my acknowledgements from the first book still stand and in addition to these are further acknowledgements related to this new book.

I would like to thank my wife, Deborah, for all her help and support through a long germination process. I am very grateful to our family friend, Catrina Donegan, who has spent much time covering for me, in the care of our children, thus allowing this and many other projects. My thanks also to my sister, Alison Smith, who helped with the first book, and with this one, has provided the working venue in the Scottish countryside to do the work, and 'fed and watered' me during it.

Also to the late Roger Houghton, Nina Martin-Brown and the late Ann Martin, literary agents without whose teaching, guidance and encouragement this book would never have been produced. To John Harrison, who was prepared to publish a book for the public on cancer. I would like to thank and to recognise the great efforts of my publishers Catharina Weijman and Alice Oven from Imperial College Press, for their dedication, tireless work and great desire to produce a well laid out and accessible book. My thanks also go to Mr Sam Abdulla, Mr Shaun Hammond, Ms Suzanne Thomas, Dr Charles Innes, Dr Tony Yardley-Jones, Mr Nigel Denby and the Rev. Gary Bradley, all of whom, over time, have shaped much of the thinking in this book. I met three people while on holiday who have been very helpful with this project, and these are Father

Vito Borgia and Joe and Carol Puttock. I would also like to thank Ms Rodena Kelman, Ms Shelby Bennett, Mrs Christine Pietraszewska, Mrs Liz Lainis and Ms Vicky Lynch for all their secretarial support without which there would be no book. My thanks also go again to Mrs Pietraszewska, Sr Catherine Gillespie, Mrs Jo Abrams and Dr Mark Bower for reading the text of *Pathways to Healing* and making many helpful suggestions. Mr Tom Lewis and Dr Bruce Barron have my gratitude for their friendship, support and introduction to my co-author, Dr Del Priore. Thanks to Dr Ben Jones for his proofreading, cross-referencing and indexing.

Many of the images appeared in two tone form originally in the *Patient Pictures* series published by Health Press and my thanks go to the publisher, Sarah Redstone, for allowing their reproduction again. My thanks also go to Laura Lee and the Board of Maggie's Centres for allowing the use of the quote in the front fly leaf.

Finally, and last, but very much not least, I would very much like to acknowledge my co-author, Dr Giuseppe Del Priore, for his help and wise advice; any mistakes and idiosyncrasies are mine!

About the Authors, Artist and Contributors

My name is Richard Smith and I am a consultant gynaecological surgeon who specialises in treating women with cancer. I was born and educated in Scotland, graduating from Glasgow University (MB, ChB). I subsequently underwent postgraduate training in the West of Scotland and London. In the late 1980s, I worked at St Mary's Hospital in London and did my thesis on the interaction of infections with cervical cancer (MD, Glasgow).

I worked for 14 years at the Chelsea and Westminster Hospital and then, with some overlap, moved to the West London Gynaecological Cancer Centre at the Hammersmith Hospital in West London. This is part of Imperial College, London and opened in 2003.

In terms of teaching, I am a Senior Lecturer at the Imperial College School of Medicine, London, UK and Adjunct Associate Professor at New York University School of Medicine.

I have had a long running interest in doctor–patient communication and have edited two series of books (The *Guide to ...* series and another series, *Patient Pictures*), which were designed to help doctors and nurses explain surgical operations to their patients. These books have sold well (approximately 240,000 books), suggesting that colleagues in both nursing and medical fields are very much interested in this area, not what you would think from looking in the press!

I have always been keen on the synthesis of 'standard' or orthodox medicine with 'complementary' medicine. This started with being taught hypnosis, practising it, and has subsequently widened out to include referring my patients for hypnotherapy, nutritional advice, acupuncture, counselling and psychotherapy. Over the last decade, I have also become convinced that although I am sure that people with some form of religious belief do not survive longer, I am sure they cope better with their cancer. For those with no religious sentiment, there are other ways of helping them to find the inner self. The synthesis of these factors allows for a truly holistic approach.

The co-author of the book is Dr Giusepe Del Priore. He is also a gynaecologist specialising in cancer treatment. He works at the Cancer Treatment Centers of America® and has a long-standing interest in doctor–patient communication. He has been a pioneer in the field of fertility sparing surgery.

The artist for the book is Ms Dee MacLean, who is one of the foremost medical artists in the world today. She has an outstanding ability to make complex anatomy look comprehensible to both doctors and patients and has a long running interest in illustrating medical problems for patients.

The Rev Gary Bradley is the Vicar of the Churches of Little Venice, London and Founder and Chairman of the Westminster Bereavement Council.

The late Mrs Mira Dharamshi, the late Mrs Patricia Walker, Mrs Gallina Dean and her husband John kindly wrote pieces as to their feelings about living with their cancer, or in John's case, his wife's cancer.

Mr Shaun Hammond is a hypnotherapist, Mr Nigel Denby is a nutritionist, Dr Tony Yardley-Jones is a consultant in occupational health, and Mr Adam Stacey-Clair is a consultant breast surgeon.

Preface

This book is designed, as the title, *Pathways to Living*, suggests, allowing you and your family ready access to all the information you require about your cancer to allow you to understand the different directions your disease may take. It should allow you to realise the breadth of possible outcomes from where you stand at the particular point in time when you buy the book, or as your disease progresses or not. This book has been written for you wherever you are in the disease, ranging from cured, to those that spend many years living with their cancer, to those who sadly die of their cancer. One of the greatest privileges working in the field of cancer care is meeting many wonderful people; very kindly, some of them have written sections of this book. It is also sadly the case that when chapters are written by people with cancers, that some of them may demise. The late Mrs Dharamshi and the late Mrs Patricia Walker were very brave and spirited women and I am grateful to them for the permission to publish their views. We do hope that by reading this book, things may be a little clearer for you and at least some worries made better.

J Richard Smith and Giuseppe Del Priore

Contents

Section I
General Information

Chapter 1

General Introduction

I have written this book in the hope of providing women who have been told that they have a cancer with accurate information that combines both orthodox medical treatments along with complementary therapies. I also hope it proves to be a valuable resource for families and supportive friends.

In comparison with 20 years ago, there are now many sources of information available to patients. These range from a plethora of 'mind, body, soul' books to innumerable websites, many of which contain highly dubious, if not frankly wrong information. In addition, you can, via 'Medline' or 'PubMed' services on the internet, access precisely the same academic papers as the doctors and nurses who care for you. Unfortunately, these papers are not written in 'patient friendly' form.

The first goal of this book is to provide you with accurate information. The second goal is that I have always believed that a combination of 'orthodox medicine' and complementary therapies, ranging from, hypnotherapy, nutritional advice, acupuncture, homeopathy, reiki, etc. allow people the best way through their diagnosis, treatment and follow up. I am a firm believer that all cancer patients deserve to hear the truth and that, contrary to popular belief, the truth, however painful, if properly imparted should not destroy hope. Below are what I would describe as the 'golden rules'.

The Golden Rules of Cancer Management

(i) Never say never. If you or your doctor believe that you are beaten before you start, then you are!

(ii) We should never say that there is nothing more that we can do for you — there always is!

(iii) The patient and the doctor are on the same team and should be working towards the same commonly understood and shared goals; quantity of life, but only if accompanied by quality.

(iv) I do not believe that spiritual peace necessarily increases longevity, but I do feel through many years of observation that those with it fare better in the cancer process than those without it. For those who have not explored this aspect of themselves, there are various other ways, some of which do not involve any religion.

How to Read the Book

This book is designed for you to read, more or less, from start to finish. It starts with four chapters that apply to all women diagnosed as having cancer. The next six chapters apply to each specific site of disease: Cervix (neck of womb), ovary, uterus (womb), vulva, breast and choriocarcinoma (cancers relating to the after-birth). You will only need to read the one relevant to you. Then follow chapters on chemotherapy and radiotherapy, which will only be relevant to those undergoing that type of treatment. The chapters on pain management may not be for you if you are not suffering from pain. Most readers will want to read the sections on complementary therapies and spiritual approaches to living with cancer.

All readers should read Gary Bradley's chapter on bereavement because this does not, as you might suppose, just relate to death, but to the whole process of coming to terms with one's diagnosis and treatment. Inevitably for all, this situation will involve some loss. At its most minor this may be the loss of feeling indestructible, which we all tend to go through life with, to loss of organs etc. this chapter is therefore a 'must read' for all.

Whenever I am explaining to my patient that they have a diagnosis of cancer, I always utilise the '4 cusp' approach, which is more fully described in Chapter 3. This seems to have proved very helpful to many women over the years, both to themselves and also in allowing them to explain to their families where they are in the process. The 4 cusp approach is really like a map for people with cancer. To facilitate its use, I suggest you draw your own '4 cusps' (see Figure 1.1) and you can mark on it where you feel yourself

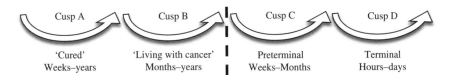

Cusp A	Cusp B	Cusp C	Cusp D
'Cured'	'Living with cancer'	Preterminal	Terminal
Weeks–years	Months–years	Weeks–Months	Hours–days

Figure 1.1   The 4 cusp approach.

to be, or alternatively, cut out the copy at the back of this book. This pictorial model demonstrates that there is hope. There is nothing more important than hope. There are three groups who have hopes: you, your family and your doctors and nurses. These hopes may vary and almost certainly will vary during the course of your disease whether you are cured or not. Hope is vital. Overall, in women with gynaecological cancer, over half are eventually cured. For those who are not cured, there is real hope of a number of years of good quality living. For those whose disease progresses, there is hope of excellent symptom control and comfort. For those who have sadly reached the end of their time, there is hope for peace and death without pain.

Concept of 'Cure'

'Cure' naturally sits very high in people's thoughts, but there are many misconceptions about what makes one cancer more curable than another. In truth, it comes down to a number of factors including which organ the cancer is in, whether it has spread from that organ, whether it is surgically removable, whether it is sensitive to chemotherapy/radiotherapy, how strong/fit the patient is, and finally and most difficult of all to know, how 'aggressive' the tumour itself is. We all know people who have had cancer that has 'just run through them' in quick order and others who are never cured of their cancer, but live with it for years. The difference between these two groups often comes down to the intrinsic aggressiveness of the tumour, something which is not easy to predict. This is why the wise doctor will avoid time spans.

You may or may not notice as you read this book that there is no mention of statistics. This is because statistics apply to groups of patients, not individual patients. They do **not** help in trying to predict what will happen to **you**. The other thing people often think statistics will help with is answering the age-old problem of 'how long have I got, doctor?' — they don't! Telling people how long they have got is a very risky thing to start doing. Quite genuinely, your doctor will rarely know the answer to this question.

The people who often struggle the most with biomedical uncertainty and the fact that statistics only apply to populations are those with a financial background and scientists: for example, physicists who are used to dealing in exact numbers, which brook no uncertainty.

I do trust that you will find reading this book useful. The chapters have been contributed to by colleagues and by three of my patients who felt very strongly that the 4 cusp approach had helped them. Sadly, Mira and Patricia, two of these three patients, have died. This partly reflects that the previous book *Pathways to Healing* was originally written in 2005. Both of these patients died after having genuinely 'lived' with their cancer for many years. They, and many others, have given me encouragement to write this book and its predecessor and all of us associated with this book earnestly hope that you find some benefit from it.

One final note: The cusps (A, B, C, D) are NOT in ANY way the same as 'stages'. The 4 cusps have proved useful to many patients; some have not found them useful, but the only people who have suffered from the concept are those who have got cusps mixed up with stages. All gynaecological cancers are staged (I, II, III, IV). There is no relationship between stages and cusps — not even a wee bit!

Chapter 2

Anatomy Overview

The Female Genital Tract

- The female genital tract includes the vulva, vagina, cervix, uterus, Fallopian tubes and ovaries.
- The vulva is the area surrounding the openings of the vagina and urethra. It includes the clitoris.
- The vagina is a muscular tube that runs from the vulva to the cervix.
- The cervix, which is sometimes called the neck of the womb, is quite firm and lies at the bottom of the uterus. During labour, it softens and then opens to allow the baby to be born.
- The uterus is a muscular organ, usually about the size of a pear, which sits in the pelvis. It is here that the foetus develops during pregnancy. The lining of the uterus is called the endometrium. This thickens during the menstrual cycle in preparation for a fertilised egg, and is shed during menstruation if the egg is not fertilised.
- The two ovaries sit on either side of the uterus. As well as producing eggs, they produce the female hormones, oestrogen and progesterone, until the menopause occurs.
- The Fallopian tubes connect the uterus to the ovaries. When an egg is released from one of the ovaries, it is collected by the Fallopian tube. Once in the tube, it may be fertilised by a sperm that has swum up from the vagina though the cervix and uterus.

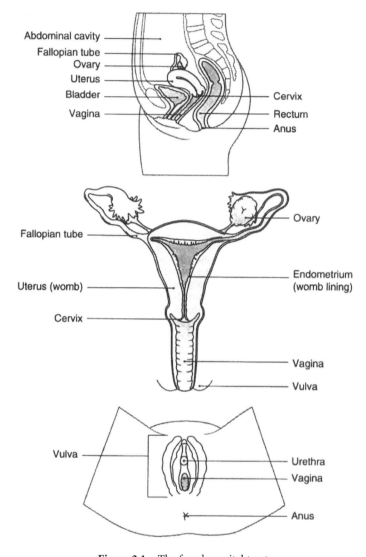

Figure 2.1   The female genital tract.

The Lymphatic System

- Lymph vessels are very fine tubes that drain the fluid, called lymph, which escapes into the body's tissues. They run next to the arteries and form a network that returns the watery fluid into the bloodstream near the heart.

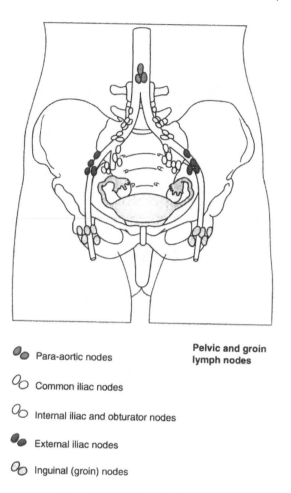

Para-aortic nodes

Pelvic and groin
lymph nodes

Common iliac nodes

Internal iliac and obturator nodes

External iliac nodes

Inguinal (groin) nodes

Figure 2.2 The lymphatic system.

- Lymph nodes, sometimes called glands, are swellings that occur near the main arteries. They act as filters for the lymph, and also have a role in the body's immune system.
- Microscopic cancer cells can escape into lymph, and can become trapped in lymph nodes. If the cells then grow, they form growths called metastases. This is one of the common ways that many cancers can spread to different parts of the body.
- Surgery for many types of cancer (including cervical, endometrial and vulval cancers) usually involves removing lymph nodes and the nearby lymph vessels.

Upper Abdominal Anatomy

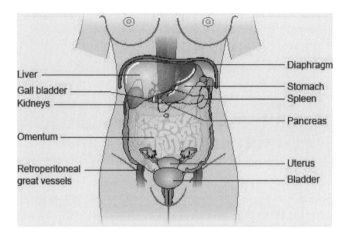

Figure 2.3   Abdominal anatomy.

Chapter 3

The 4 Cusp Approach
to Cancer Care

My colleagues, medical oncologist Dr Mark Bower and specialist nurse Sr Catherine Gillespie, and I have developed this approach to patient care over many years of sitting in clinics explaining to patients where they are with their cancer, not just in physical terms, but conceptually in relation to their cancer and their life expectancy and its quality.

IT IS VITALLY IMPORTANT TO STATE THAT THE '4 CUSPS' (A–D) BEAR <u>NO</u> RELATIONSHIP TO THE FOUR STAGES (I, II, III AND IV) OF CANCER.

Stages refer to how far a cancer has spread and are described in detail in Chapters 6–10.

Perhaps the two most important aspects of the 4 cusp pictorial model are the action of folding it down the central line and the 'circle' aimed at in both Cusps A and B. I believe that being able to fold the paper and thus dispatch Cusp C and D to being 'out of sight', coupled with the powerful image of a circle suggesting 'holism', are the model's strongest features. If you can, it would be good if you could draw the 4 cusps on a piece of paper as shown here (Figure 3.1) (or cut out the one provided at the end of this book):

This pictorial representation or 'map' to having cancer has seemed to resonate with patients and their families. I think that, perhaps, symbols can represent concepts that are difficult with language. In the words of

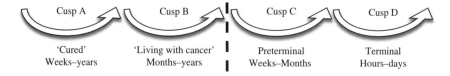

Figure 3.1   The 4 cusp approach diagram.

St Thomas Aquinas, 'man cannot understand without images'. A PhD student did a project to assess the 4 cusp model, which showed that it resonated well with patients and their families. When you are told of your cancer diagnosis, you will probably jump to the conclusion that you have been given a 'death sentence'. You will almost certainly immediately forget the remainder of the consultation, only remembering the diagnosis itself. The first thing I am able to tell the vast majority of my patients is that they are not in Cusps C and D, but either in Cusp A or B, and thus we can fold the paper down the dotted line and that we can literally put Cusps C and D out of the way. You may find it helpful to do this right now with the 4 cusps you have drawn. All of us are different and every cancer is different, but it is important in the first instance to be aware that *over 50% of gynaecological tumours are cured in the long term*. The 'death sentence' outlook is just not true for most people. At your first consultation for a suspected or confirmed cancer, you will be given an outline of the timetable as to when investigations will be done and if, when and where your surgery will take place. You will be told that full results, including exactly how far your cancer has progressed, will be known by a specific date. At that time, it will be possible to talk far more accurately about your outlook and prospects. The specific timetable to confirm the diagnosis, undertake any surgery and obtain the results of the analysis of the removed cancer should take two to four weeks approximately, although this may be quicker (one week) for some and slower (five to six weeks) for others.

When all the information is available, your doctor will wish to talk to you, perhaps on the ward or more often in a consultation room. Your doctor will tell you your results and what these will mean for you. My own golden rule here is to impart the truth, and nothing but the truth, in as gentle a fashion as I can. More and more doctors are receiving training in communication and it is likely that the appropriate language will be used.

Not surprisingly, it is known that this type of doctor–patient communication is the greatest cause of anxiety for doctors in training. Inevitably, however much training people have, some prove to be better at it than others. It is a facet of human nature that all of us prefer to tell people good news and most of us generally shy away from bad news, either giving or receiving it. All the professional training that goes into creating doctors cannot, nor for that matter should it, negate these emotions. We all know that in our daily lives we meet people who we describe as 'sensitive' or 'insensitive'; this applies as much to doctors as to their patients. It is also true that in terms of personality type, the person who chooses to become a surgeon tends to the more self-confident and at the aggressive end of the spectrum, which are not features that always predispose to 'touchy feely' behaviour, but they do, however, tend to make for bold and effective surgeons. That is not to suggest that these surgeons are uncaring or that there are not plenty of sensitive surgeons in the world. I know many years ago, I was required to have some fairly big surgery: I went to somebody who could not be described as 'touchy feely' but wow, could they operate. That was the most important thing for me in that circumstance.

The other factor that comes into play is the 'dynamic' of the relationship between two individuals. Forgetting the medical situation, we all know that when we walk into a party where we don't know many people that, in general, we'll get along OK with most people; sometimes we'll become good friends with somebody we meet, and occasionally, we might marry that good friend. The opposite sometimes happens where we meet somebody we truly dislike. It is worth remembering that they probably feel the same way about us! The nature of human relationships is that although 'we feel for ourselves', these feelings are usually mutual and reciprocated.

The professional relationship between patient and doctor is designed to remove the extremes described above (doctors who hate or marry their patients tend to end up being struck off the medical register), but it doesn't detract from the fact that we all still get on better with some people than with others. The good doctor should have the sensitivity and capacity to get on with the vast majority of his/her patients.

A commonly asked question is, 'How long have I got?' No doctor is likely, if he/she has any sense, to answer this question directly, since they do not and cannot know the answer. They are much more likely to answer using a variant of the 4 cusp approach to cancer care. This is patient-centred and allows you to see where you are with your disease. I have spent many years drawing pictures for patients showing them which operation they were going to have. Rarely has the picture been taken away for future reference. This may be because of the quality of my artwork or it may be that people get the message. On the other hand, the 4 cusp diagram has been taken away by numerous patients who have found it very helpful, both for themselves and to assist in further dialogue with their families.

This has proved to be a very useful method of communicating concepts of cure, living and dying with cancer, and I will now explain it in more detail. This concept will be used throughout the book, so please read this section with care. It may be helpful to bookmark it.

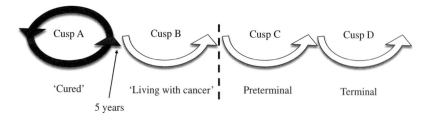

Figure 3.2   Cusp A, 'cured'.

The first cusp (Cusp A, Figure 3.2) probably applies to you from the time of your first visit to the clinic, when your surgeon gives the likely diagnosis and discusses with you the plan of action to determine how advanced your cancer is and hopefully how to remove it. Your surgeon can usually be confident before surgery that they can either cure the cancer with surgery or, failing that, at least put you in the best jumping-off point for further treatment. For some patients, the best approach may be to use chemotherapy first and then follow it with surgery. If surgery is the plan, your surgeon will feel that the cancer is resectable to the point of you being made either potentially curable, or capable of remission. What you need is an honest appraisal of the possibilities along with a plan of action. This should include the date of surgery, length of time in hospital and when the final results of tests will be available. All tissue samples go to the laboratory for testing (histopathology and cytopathology) and it is these results that absolutely determine the diagnosis and how advanced the cancer is. It is almost always possible to achieve these results within two to six weeks of your first visit to the clinic. You and your family will therefore have a good idea of where you stand by a specific date in the near future.

Your surgeon will explain how much your cancer has spread (or not). This will determine whether you require no other treatment because you are thought to be cured or whether you may need radiotherapy or chemotherapy or a combination of the two, either just to be on the safe side or because a cure is not likely without them. In addition, it is at this point that it may be suggested that you have chemotherapy before further assessment as to whether your surgeon may be able to remove remaining tumours at a future date, usually after three to four months.

In general, if surgery alone is the only treatment, you will be told that you are highly likely to be cured. This, however, can only be confirmed by the passage of time and the longer all remains well, the higher is the likelihood that you are cured. Your surgeon will rightly be buoyant and optimistic with you. He/she will however explain that there is a small chance of the cancer coming back (a relapse) and you will need to be seen in the clinic for a number of years. You fall into the following 4 cusp picture. You may find it helpful at this point to copy this onto your drawing of the 4 cusps.

The following are case histories of patients, all of which directly relate to women I have looked after over the last few years and which illustrate the 4 cusp approach.

Patient 1

A 35-year-old woman is referred to the gynaecology oncology clinic with bleeding after sex and her general practitioner (GP) suspects she may have a cervical cancer (remember the vast majority of women with bleeding after sex do not have cervical cancer). The woman has completed her family. When the woman is examined, there is a small cervical cancer with no evidence of spread elsewhere. It is explained that she has a cancer, which has only developed recently, and that she is likely to be highly curable by surgery alone. The patient is then admitted for an examination in theatre with the patient asleep, in other words under general anaesthetic. This allows for proper assessment of (see page 65) the tumour without any discomfort to the woman. This confirms that surgery is the best way forward and a few days later, she has a special type of hysterectomy (see pages 71 and 72). One week after that, all the results are available.

Option 1

It is shown that the cancer has been completely removed and that there is no spread to the lymph nodes (glands). This means that the woman is presumed cured, i.e. she remains at **Cusp A** (Figure 3.2). It is only after 5 years that she can know she is truly cured.

Option 2

The tumour is completely removed but the cancer has spread to three lymph glands. It is explained that these cancers do, if they are going to spread, tend to go to the lymph glands first. The lymph glands normally help to protect the body from things like infection, by acting as a kind of filter. When there is a cancer, they also filter out cancer cells and prevent spread more widely around the body, so that although it is better not to have spread to the lymph glands, they have still done their job by preventing more extensive spread. In this woman's case, the lymph glands have been removed, but because they have tumours in them, she requires further treatment in the form of chemo-radiotherapy. It is explained that this being overcautious is the usual approach ('belt and braces/suspenders', i.e. if you don't want your trousers to fall down ever, you wear both). This patient has entered **Cusp B** (see Figure 3.3); she is probably cured, but may not be, and is therefore 'living with her cancer', certainly not dying of it.

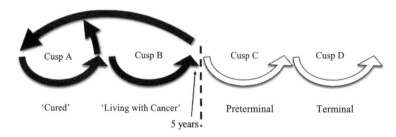

Figure 3.3   The 'living with cancer' circle. At five years, if all is well, she moves to the 'cured' circle, and then at that point the inverted commas around cured can be removed.

Sometimes I will suggest that the patient looks in the mirror in clinic, and see herself: it is completely obvious that she is not looking at someone who is dying because she looks normal! In terms of the 4 cusp model, this is shown below. You may find it helpful to copy this onto your '4 cusp' drawing.

Patient 2

A 55-year-old woman goes to see her doctor since she has noticed swelling in her tummy over the last few weeks. She is referred to the specialist gynaecological cancer surgeon and they agree that she seems to have a growth in her ovary. It is explained that she may have a benign tumour or it may be malignant. Either way, she requires an ultrasound scan, a magnetic resonance imaging (MRI) scan, a computed tomography (CT) scan and some blood tests. The results of these tests suggest that she has a cancer within her ovary, but that it appears to be confined to one ovary with no spread (this is called stage Ia, see page 83). It is explained to the woman that she requires surgery in the form of a hysterectomy and removal of both ovaries (see pages 89 and 90), lymph nodes (glands) and a fatty structure in the abdomen called the omentum (see also pages 89 and 90). Very few patients (unless they are a doctor themselves) have heard of the omentum. The omentum is a fatty structure that moves around the abdomen to where there is trouble. For example, in the past (pre-1900), before surgery was widely available, if you had an appendicitis, you were quite likely to die; however, you could be saved by your omentum, which would move around the appendix and stop the infection from spreading. The omentum also moves itself around ovarian cancers to prevent them from spreading, but unfortunately, in the process, cancers easily spread to the omentum itself, hence it requires to be removed. The authors do not know of anyone who has missed their omentum once it's out! One week later, the patient undergoes the planned operation.

Option 1

A tumour is removed, which is in one ovary alone (see Figure 3.2). The patient requires no further treatment and is presumed cured; in other words, she is in **Cusp A**, as shown in Figure 3.2. You may wish to draw this on your '4 cusps'. Note that she can only know she is cured after 5 years of remission have elapsed.

Option 2

The patient is found to have cancer in both of her ovaries and fluid containing cancerous cells in her abdomen (see Figure 3.3). She requires chemotherapy; she has entered **Cusp B**. It is explained that she has good prospects for cure, but that only time will confirm this; she is 'living with cancer'. However, five years later, she has shown no sign of tumour recurrence and therefore, has returned to the 'cured' circle (**Cusp A**); this is shown in Figure 3.3.

Option 3

The patient is found at surgery to have disseminated (or widespread) cancer all over her abdomen. The technical term for how far the cancer has spread is the 'stage' of the cancer; in other words, how advanced it is, and in this case, it is called Stage III (see page 84). She is now in **Cusp B**. It is explained that chemotherapy can be expected to work, but it cannot be said with certainty how great the effect will be. Some cancers respond extremely well to chemotherapy, some poorly, and the majority somewhere in between. Thus, it may not produce a cure; however, the longer it keeps the tumour under control, the better it is, both directly in terms of possible cure and indirectly, since the tumour that responds to chemotherapy in the

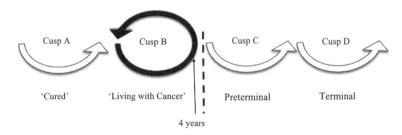

Figure 3.4   When there is recurrence at 4 years, she goes back to the start of Cusp B and remains 'living with cancer'.

first instance is more likely to respond to a second course of treatment. Thus, there are three scenarios here:

(i) Excellent response and at five years, the patient has no sign of tumour recurrence; thus, she has returned to **Cusp A** (Figure 3.3).

(ii) A good response is made and the patient remains well for four years, at which point she develops recurrence of her cancer. She is treated again with either more surgery or the same chemotherapy as before with good prospects of a similar 2–4 year response again. Thus, she remains in **Cusp B** (Figure 3.4).

(iii) A poor response is made with the cancer recurring four months later. This patient has now entered **Cusp C** (Figure 3.5).

This woman has very little chance of cure and has therefore entered the preterminal phase of her illness. She is informed that she is unlikely to be cured and that she has a limited time left, which may be weeks or may be months, but is unlikely to be longer than this. She is informed that there are plenty of treatment options still available, and although they are designed mainly to enhance quality of life, they may also extend it. These types of treatment are called palliative care and may include pain relief, treatment of constipation or diarrhoea and many other things that are described in Chapter 13.

Healing — What Role Can Faith Play?

Three of my patients kindly agreed to write a piece for this part of the book because they felt strongly that they had very much benefited from

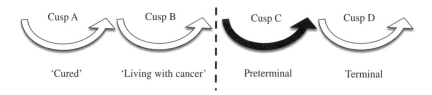

Figure 3.5 Cusp C, 'preterminal'.

the concept of 'living with cancer'. Sadly, Mira and Patricia, two of the three patients who wrote for the original book, *Pathways to Healing*, have died. With respect to Mira's piece, her wishes have been followed, namely of publishing the piece unedited. This was her specific request and I have to say that while the sentiments expressed in her piece are very flattering to one of the authors (JRS), I suggested to her that they would be better not to appear in print! Mira told me that she wished them printed as she had written them and I have therefore followed her wishes and not exercised any editorial control! With respect to Galina's text, Galina has accessed many complementary therapies and her text is unedited. It is important to say that all of the opinions mentioned may not accord with the views of the authors.

Recollections of Mira Dharamshi

I remember clearly the day I was told I had ovarian cancer. My first thoughts were: why me? What have I done wrong? Not that I was a stranger to cancer, having lost a younger sister to the disease several years earlier. She was diagnosed with leukaemia, so I was well versed with the 'Big C'. I had seen her go through the trauma of chemotherapy and radiotherapy. But only in hindsight do I realise that I experienced for the first time the role that faith could play in helping one cope with the illness. At the time, I would ask my sister cynically: where is God now that you need him most? Her reply was always that God was giving her the strength to go through this. In my wisdom then, I required proof of God's existence because if he existed, why wasn't he helping her?

Proof of course is beside the point. The essential issue for me now is 'faith'. It is, I believe, the driving force behind my ability to persevere through my cancerous journey. Faith can take many guises: faith in God or some sort of spiritual plane; faith in oneself, one's consultant, one's family, friends, etc. My own faith takes many forms.

My faith can certainly be summed up as a conventional belief in God. But my consultant, medical treatment, and support and help from people around me also play an important role in my wellbeing.

I felt extremely angry watching my sister go through her illness. But her courage and faith that she would ultimately get better never wavered. Unfortunately, she passed away a few months later. I promised myself that if I ever developed cancer, I wouldn't go through what she had, that is, the gruelling treatment in a bid to extend the amount of time I had. How wrong was I, as here I am, after many years of living with and tackling the disease, telling my tale.

I did want to die as soon as I was told that I had cancer. My reasoning was that I could escape the pain and suffering through early release. After receiving news about my illness from the doctor, I remember vividly standing at a bus stop. It was New Year's Eve, the streets were full of Christmas decoration, crowds were rushing about and it was bitterly cold. I didn't know whom to talk to. My husband was at work; should I tell him immediately or wait until I knew the prognosis? I stood zombie-like, numb — my mind scheming and plotting some sort of plan on what to do next. Having no other immediate family in London except for my husband, I felt alone. I wanted to spare him the anguish I felt seeing my sister go through her illness. I would be dead soon, I thought. But what would happen to my husband and my nieces? And, in the meantime, how would I tell my father, who lived in Kenya? The shock, I thought, may kill him.

As it turned out, I was spared the decision of telling my father news of my illness as he passed away in the interim period before my consultant's appointment. I also refrained from telling my family and made an excuse not to attend my father's funeral. Understandably, the family considered this odd as I was viewed as his favourite daughter and supported him financially.

I decided I would visit the consultant alone. After all, I knew exactly what I wanted: in the event that the disease was substantial, I didn't want any treatment at all — such was my lack of faith in myself, medicine and ultimately, in God.

The first appointment was a mixed bag; the consultant was very smart, looked very young, and I was told by my gynaecologist that he was the best. And now I know he is; nevertheless, he was very amenable to talk to. He explained in detail that I had a lump on my inferior vena cava and a 'mass' on my ovary. A hysterectomy was therefore on the cards.

I was devastated by the prognosis. I could feel tears rolling down my cheeks despite the fact I had promised myself I wouldn't break down. But I was comfortable talking to him, describing how I felt and telling him about my sister. I didn't want any treatment if the cancer was widespread and definitely no chemotherapy. After lengthy discussions with my consultant, it was agreed that he would undertake an exploratory operation to assess the situation, and then discuss the way forward. He agreed, though, to respect my wishes and would do whatever I decided.

The trials that followed over the next seven years included: five operations; three sets of chemotherapy of carboplatin, Taxol, radio-therapy; contracting septicaemia; losing my hair, accompanied by fun and games with wigs and turbans; and, unrelated to the illness, breaking my right arm, which resulted in the insertion of two metal pins and a plate in my elbow; and having a younger brother gunned down by a bank robber in Nairobi. In addition, I almost lost the one thing I continue to enjoy immensely — my job — after the company underwent one of the most acrimonious and hostile take-overs ever fought in the city of London. Being told my job no longer existed was an enormous shock and filled me with the dread of having to find another job — an almost impossible task, I thought, given my medical history. For the time being, I have managed to secure a position in the marketing department, but for how long?

At one point, a nurse had said to me: 'I have seen you down in the dumps many times, but you always pick yourself up. I don't know how you do it.' Similarly, I don't know what drives me to per-severe, despite the difficulties associated with the illness as well as life's hardships. Sometimes, I wonder if I am from another planet and am an alien; it is just not possible with all of these things hap-pening. It seems like a James Bond movie drama; despite going through hell and fire, you come out smiling.

My colleagues have sometimes joked that the sickness record in the office has dropped as a result of my attitude. If I can make it to the office whilst undergoing chemotherapy, for example, they can also show up for a day's work even when they have minor ailments. But I don't necessarily entertain a positive attitude — despite others' belief to the contrary — and have never been afraid of dying. My aim is to maintain a good quality of life, not to live at any cost and be a burden to my family.

It is difficult to express what drives me; perhaps it is just sheer determination. I manage to hold a full-time job, tackling the daily commute into and out of London by changing two trains, and often work late into the evening. I have continued working daily while having chemo and, at one point, had to contend with one arm in plaster for eight weeks.

Waiting for a bus one day, I overheard a lady say: 'O' it was God sent'. This struck a chord with me. God may not touch you directly, but someone or something in your life can give you strength — be it your general faith, husband, a friend, a nurse, or one's faith in a consultant.

The thing I most remember is my consultant saying to me that I should allow him to help rid me of cancer. He also expressed hope that I could avoid the thing I dreaded most — chemotherapy. His words proved powerful. He said he would give his sister, for example, exactly the same advice if she were in the same position as me. This ultimately prompted me to change my mind and agree to have the exploratory operation and the subsequent treatment. Here was someone I didn't know, wasn't related to me, but cared for me and wanted to help make me better. He listened to my concerns, explained in detail that I was in the so-called second cusp — that is, living with cancer — and exactly how he planned to treat me. I would never ask him how long I had as I think no one can give you that guarantee.

The upshot is that deep in my inner self, the faith I have in God gives me strength. Many a times, I ask God: 'Why am I being punished? What have I done?' I consider myself to be a good person, but not a saint. I often recall what my mother used to say when questioned about God and different aspects of worship: 'I am your mother, a wife to your father, an aunt, a grandmother, a daughter, but I am only one person. God also has numerous names, but is only one. No one has seen him; though we all believe that he exists and have faith that he will provide strength in times of need.'

Travelling to work each day — which takes roughly over one hour — I recite my prayers. I pray for world peace, for all who are sick and need help, pray that God gives me strength to cope with my illness and that I do not suffer or prove to be a burden to my family towards the end of my illness. I also pray that, whenever it arrives, I meet a peaceful end.

Recollections of Patricia Walker

I must have been living with cancer a long while before finding out. I did not even connect a series of rather vague symptoms, ranging from repeated bouts of cystitis to an increasingly swollen stomach. When I appeared, to me at least, to look in an advanced state of pregnancy, the duty GP simply asked if I had considered liposuction. Eventually, sudden breathtakingly sharp stomach pains sent me to hospital.

The diagnosis of Stage III ovarian cancer, and the subsequent removal of 'a tumour the size of a rugby ball' two days before my 64th birthday, was a complete and potentially devastating surprise. I had no real idea of what it meant and found it hard at first to absorb the information I was given. Happily, almost as big a surprise was the number of ways that the hospital team helped me to cope. It was important that from the very beginning, like others on the gynaecological ward, I was treated not just as a patient, or a case, or a hospital number, but as a named individual whose personal concerns and preferences were sought, considered and taken into account.

Doctors have something in common with airline pilots. They have to strike a balance between being seriously knowledgeable and competent and being reassuringly relaxed, and to do this without sounding so laid back and blasé that their passengers (patients) expect the worst. I liked the tone of voices at the Chelsea and Westminster (C&W) very much: realistic, warm, comforting, professional and personal.

The gynaecology consultant was extraordinarily generous with his time, explaining the diagnosis, proposed operation, likely treatment and intended outcome. He drew annotated diagrams which, if not high art, very effectively communicated the facts and have been invaluable for later reference. The oncologist knew that my husband had been a patient at the C&W and thoughtfully took this into account with options for treatment. The supporting professionals also communicated well, listening and responding to what they were being asked. The different disciplines involved in my treatment seemed to work as a cooperative and accessible team and I felt, at least temporarily, a part of that team and sharing the same focus.

My main reaction to all this was to feel personal responsibility for my progress and only a distant academic interest in discouraging statistics. I was not avoiding reality, but deciding that all available energy would be needed for getting better.

Landmarks became very important. At first, they were small and frequent: getting out of bed, coping without a catheter, having a shower (thank you, Sharon!), walking down the corridor. Everyone was substantial reassurance that things were progressing as predicted. Later, each chemotherapy treatment was a landmark, with the CA-125 blood test result assuming enormous significance and regularly demonstrating progress.

The biggest (to me) early landmark provided a salutary lesson: use landmarks, but don't depend on them. It was the joint oncology/gynaecology review booked before I left hospital. When neither consultant was available at the appointment (for very good reasons), the disappointment was like a physical blow.

By contrast, there was a positive physical effect from the consistent kindness, consideration, competence and cheerfulness found throughout the hospital. The medical day unit where chemotherapy is administered is a particularly good example. Chemotherapy is not normally the jolliest way to pass a day, but the staff have created a unique atmosphere and relationships with their customers, as well as their colleagues, that inspire confidence and give invaluable practical and psychological support and inspired confidence.

The first chemotherapy treatment, with carboplatin and Taxol, had three particular side effects. One was hair loss, which proved much less of a physical and emotional problem than anticipated. A wig, a knitted hat and two silk scarves covered every eventuality.

The hair started growing back as soon as the chemotherapy finished. This was totally fascinating for my small granddaughters. My hair was the same colour — not always the case — but initially Afro-curly; then looser curls; then wavy as before chemotherapy; then straight.

A second side effect was the constipation, which did not go away. Experimenting with a variety of prescription medicines identified the most suitable, with prunes or prune juice and dried figs playing a major supporting role. The medical day unit nurses were very familiar with the problem and their experience was invaluable.

A third side effect was neuropathy: numbness of the fingers and feet. Once the chemotherapy had finished, the fingers recovered fairly quickly; dipping them in alternatively hot and cold water helped. The balls of the feet and the toes did not. The nurses suggested treatment by a hospital-based reflexologist, a trained therapist who volunteered her services one day a week. Reflexology every two or three weeks restored a great deal of feeling and made walking safer and more confident. It was also wonderfully relaxing. Other treatments available included massage and relaxation classes. While complementary therapies have their place and undoubtedly have been helpful to me, and how and where they are given is important. It proved quite impossible to learn relaxation techniques in an airless room on a carpet sprinkled with biscuit crumbs and discarded food wrappings.

Away from the hospital, I had two opportunities for reiki treatments. The first one was remarkable. A warm glow over my stomach, although the practitioner had not touched me, produced complete relaxation and a sense of peaceful wellbeing. The other had the opposite effect. The second practitioner talked nonstop throughout about her own activities and plans for practising other therapies which left me twanging with tension.

During the first chemotherapy, both my neighbour and sister-in-law had asked for remote spiritual healing for me. It was as important that they felt they were doing something to help as that I felt supported by them in this way. Coping with cancer can be as hard or harder for family and friends as for the patient, especially when they feel powerless. Individuals found so many ways to help: scouring the internet for information, recommending books they had enjoyed, sharing funny newspaper cuttings, cheerful telephone calls, not just inviting me to lunch or dinner, but thoughtfully arranging transport too, and encouraging business as usual in terms of work.

Work has been as important as treatment. It has confirmed that my brain still works, that people still want to use it and that I still have something important to contribute. Getting paid is a very welcome endorsement of this. Equally important, however, has been the reassurance of a variety of charitable and other organisations, which are just as eager for involvement and advice, even if more may be done by e-mail or over the telephone than previously. Two new appointments while living with cancer have been particularly welcome, as both organisations were fully aware of the circumstances when they employed me.

How much people want to know differs. Sometimes 'how are you?' expects a fairly detailed answer about treatment and response to it. For others, 'doing well' may be as much as they feel they can cope with. My daughter wants to know everything and from the first, I made sure my medical notes said she was to be told everything.

It was ten months before I started chemotherapy again, this time with Caelyx. There was no hair loss, no sickness, and no side effects, which suggested to me that it was having no effect. It was stopped after three cycles. Subsequently, the CA-125 tests demonstrated an improvement.

It was at this stage that a group of close friends organised a marvellous event. Twenty female friends sat down to a lunch for which they had brought food, wine, flowers and much crockery. Many had never met each other before (but a lot of them have met again since). The premise was that all the compliments that are paid at funerals and memorial services are not heard by the one person they directly concern. So why not arrange a lunch where friends can pay their compliments in person? My daughter thought it sounded morbid, but in the event she found it an incredibly happy, noisy and uplifting occasion — as I did — and she recorded the proceedings on video to prove it. It was a tremendously supportive and confidence inspiring day; and confidence — in the hospital, professionals, treatment, advice, information and people — is the most important single aid to living with cancer.

Nearly three years after my operation, I was due to start chemotherapy again. The start was delayed: firstly, because I was taking antibiotics for an infection; then for no apparent reason, despite a very high CA-125 result. It was a couple of months before affected patients were told that the National Health Service (NHS) had decreed that all gynaecological cancers were to be treated at cancer centres and the C&W had been designated a unit, not a centre. We were compulsorily evicted from the hospital and from the team we knew and trusted. This was inevitably demoralising.

The cancer centre has struggled to cope with the sudden influx of new patients at different stages of diagnosis and treatment. There were inevitable delays for the first appointment. It was months before chemotherapy started again, by then with a bigger job to do. Fortunately, after the first two cycles the CA-125 has fallen dramatically and although the CT scan appears to show that the tumours have not shrunk, they are not noticeably larger.

In the bigger, busier specialist cancer centre, there is not the same close team and continuity of staff. Although no doubt in excellent hands, those hands are constantly changing and it is much harder to establish relationships, not helped by the fact that the surgeon and oncologist are now in different centres. It will therefore take a while to recover the confidence which is so essential to living with cancer.

Recollections of Galina Dean

So Far So Good: One Person's Fight against Ovarian Cancer.

In September 2002, at the age of 38, after six weeks of unexplained abdominal pain, I was diagnosed with Stage IV ovarian cancer. I had always thought of myself as a healthy person, with the exception of the fact that I had a benign ovarian cyst and the relevant ovary removed in 1982. I had yearly ultrasound tests and internal examinations. I felt that my health was good. I exercised regularly and had a good diet. My parents were both healthy and I did not imagine that anything serious could happen to me.

Looking back, I remember exactly when the symptoms started — it was in the middle of July 2002. My husband, John, and I had just returned from vacation in France. I constantly had a problem with constipation over 4–5 years, but it got worse when we came back from vacation. I had taken laxatives from time to time over a long period, but increased the dosage after the holiday. The pain I experienced with any bowel movement was unimaginable. I also started having stomach spasms after eating and my abdomen became swollen.

I originally thought that this was a consequence of food poisoning in France. However, after a week the problem did not go away and so I went to see my local GP. He sent me home, saying that it was certainly food poisoning, and that I would be fine in a week or so.

I did not get better and went to see him again after ten days. By this time my abdomen was noticeably swollen and I was wearing the biggest trousers I had in my wardrobe. He said, 'I cannot see any problem, you look fine!' I said to him, 'What do I have to do as I am having intense pain.' He gave me pain killers and sent me home!

Within 4–5 days, I was forced to queue up to see another doctor at the same practice who, after an internal examination, organised an ultrasound test for me at the C&W Hospital.

The girl in the ultrasound room told me that there was nothing suspicious, and that I should come back in 2–3 months' time. At the time, I asked her to look a little higher up in the stomach area; however, she refused, saying that in the instruction from the GP, the only request had been for an ultrasound of the ovary! This was exactly one week before I was diagnosed with OVARIAN CANCER!

The pain became more and more intense. I couldn't eat anything; my stomach was distended as if I was pregnant. I again went back to the original GP and begged him to organise a blood test. He said that this was not necessary as he now knew exactly what the problem was. He sent me to the Lydia Clinic, which at the time did not mean anything to me, and I went along with no misgivings. The pain was so bad that I could hardly think about anything.

However, imagine my surprise when I found out that this was a venereal disease clinic!

My husband was very angry when I told him what had happened and attended the meeting the next day with the GP. We both insisted that he take a blood sample, which he finally agreed to do.

That night I had a high temperature, had not eaten for 3–4 days and had difficulty breathing. The next morning, I could not wait any more and asked my husband to take me to the hospital as an emergency case. The Chelsea & Westminster Hospital (C&W) is no more than 10–15 minutes' drive from our house and as we were driving there, my GP called to say that he had the blood test results, which were very bad, and that we should go immediately to see him. We did this and he gave us the paperwork for me to be admitted to the C&W as an emergency case. There is an important point to be made here which is that **if you suspect a problem that does not go away, be active and do not be 'fobbed' off by your GP!**

In the worst case, you can always pay for a blood test and take the results to your doctor. If I had known what I know now, I would have had a CA-125 test (tumour marker) done immediately. At the time I did not know that this kind of test existed. The normal range for this test is 0–23. At the time of my admittance, my 'score' was 2,700!

I was admitted to C&W on a Friday and finally, after a full day of tests, I was given an MRI scan. I was then kept in hospital over the weekend whilst they drained the fluid which had been distending my abdomen.

Finally, the initial nightmare ended and on the Monday, Mr Smith, the gynaecological surgeon, came to see me and told me that I had tumours on my ovary, my omentum and my stomach. He said that they had tested the fluid with which I was swollen to find that it was full of cancer cells. I also had fluid in my lungs.

Even though 'cancer' was the last name I wanted to hear, I felt some relief that my illness at last had a name and I could start receiving treatment, and that maybe, one day, I would start feeling better. I believed in Mr Smith, his kind eyes radiated confidence, and I knew that this man would help me.

John was there with me. No need to describe our feelings. We could not believe what was happening. This was something unreal. At this stage, all I knew about cancer was that people died from it.

'Am I dying?' was my first question to Mr Smith. 'How long do I have?' He explained that I was not in the terminal stage, so I had some time. Then for my second question, I asked Mr Smith to give me survival statistics for my situation. He said, 'I will give you statistics if you want, but everybody is an individual case. Most women with the disease are over the age of 55'.

I wanted to know anyway. The answer was that only one in three to four women in the sample survived beyond five years. I could not believe what I was hearing. I was not ready. When Mr Smith's team left the room, John and I hugged one another and started crying together...

I felt that it was my fault that, because of my illness, I felt that I was letting him down, I was letting our relationship down and I was letting my parents and all my friends down.

That night, I pulled myself together. I thought I had no right to let so many people down, so many people I loved; I could not let them suffer. I thought, 'I will fight and I will survive'.

On Mr Smith's recommendation and that of Dr Bower from the C&W oncology department, I had four rounds of chemotherapy (Taxol/carboplatin) before my operation. I had been warned about all the side effects. The worst one was that I was going to lose my hair, my long, blond hair, which I had always been proud of. I was going to lose all of it...

I felt weak and helpless after the first round of chemo, I presumed in my case it was because I was having the treatment straight after being in hospital on a drip and 'nil by mouth' for a week, so I was pretty weak already. For the first 3–4 days after chemo, I lost weight, 1–1.5 kilos every day. My normal weight had been 50 kilos for the last 15 years and with the fluid accumulation it had reached 54. I felt very weak and tired, sometimes not to be able to lift a glass of water. It was pretty unpleasant, I felt like an invalid. I decided at that point to do something positive!

Next morning I asked John to take me to the Ki Energy Institute in London, NW1. A close girl friend strongly recommended this approach. She had benefited enormously from their treatments and had been using them to boost her general health for three years. The method is derived from 6,000 year-old Taoist tradition originating in South Korea. I could hardly walk; John almost carried me from the car.

After 2–3 hours of treatment, I felt much better, walking by myself and felt strong enough to walk in the park for two hours. From that point, I went there every day. For the first two weeks, John drove me, and after that I was able to drive myself… I started to feel better from the first day and the pain lessened. I did not take this for granted. I remember on bad days when I said to my husband, 'If only this pain will go away, I will not ask for anything else, I will be the happiest person in the world!'

My weight stabilised around 48 kilos. The pain went completely and my stomach became flat again. I restarted a gentle exercise regime just to tone my muscles. I bought a lot of books on the subject of cancer to investigate as much as possible. My first real inspiration came from the book, *The Cancer Battle*, about a woman who was sent home to die with progressive breast cancer. Twelve years on, she is still alive, healthy and happy!

Reading this book, I realised that one has to take responsibility for one's own body. The key statement in the book was, 'Your body has the ability to completely heal itself of any disease…all it needs is your assistance'. From this point, the real action started.

A reverse osmosis filter was installed in our house. Pure water is very important and with ovarian cancer I wanted to make sure that any oestrogen and any oestrogen mimics were removed from the water I was drinking. I started to make fresh juice 3–4 times per day (carrot, apple, fennel, beetroot and wheat grass); this helps the body detoxify. The concentrated amount of vitamins, minerals and enzymes in very fresh juice assimilate quickly and easily into one's blood. I stopped drinking coffee and tea, switching to herbal infusions/teas. I gave up alcohol and stopped eating sugar, wheat, milk products and meat…

As soon as we found a sensible wig, I had my hair cut off, (I still keep it as a souvenir), because the worst nightmare would have been to see my hair on the pillow every morning. I realised very quickly that I had to make the best of the situation I was in, otherwise I would go mad. My wig was not cheap, but I rationalised this with the idea that I was going to save on shampoo, conditioner, haircuts, etc. for several months.

The rest of the rounds of chemotherapy went pretty well for me. I felt OK and managed to lead a more or less normal life, going out from time to time and going to the gym. I had been involved in the property market in a small way and was able to resume this activity.

I had my fourth round of chemo just before my birthday in November 2002. My CA-125 count was 32. On the 2nd December 2002, Mr Smith performed a hysterectomy and also removed my omentum. After Christmas I had to face another four rounds of chemo; this finished in March 2003. Between rounds 6 and 7 of chemotherapy I visited the Paracelsus Klinic in Switzerland with my husband. I had talked to them a few weeks before and they had strongly suggested that this was a good time to be treated by them. Their approach is based on biological medicine, but at the same time, they try to work together with orthodox treatments. I had a very busy schedule and they performed many different tests on me. I was given a large box of pills to take every day with very little explanation.

I found it pretty stressful not to understand what I was being asked to put in my body. As I had a very low red blood cell count, I could not take all the treatments at that time. They therefore suggested that I come back after the last round of chemo, but it was a very, very expensive two weeks.

I wanted to make a clear plan of what I was going to do when the chemo finished. One of our friends gave a book entitled, *Everything you need to know to help you beat Cancer* by a biochemist, Chris Woollams. It is one of the most useful books that I have read. He also gave me a copy of the magazine that Chris Woollams edits called, *ICON*. I immediately subscribed to this magazine and have found it to be very useful.

The book contains a lot of information about how to help yourself recover after chemotherapy and tumour removal operations. I was shocked by the news that almost all cancer sufferers are very toxic, their bodies can be very acidic and can also have a high level of parasites, viruses and/or yeast. So my first step was to check these things. I had all of them!

I met a woman at the Ki Energy Institute who had been diagnosed with melanoma three years ago. She had refused any orthodox treatment and had undertaken a course of natural healing instead. She recommended me to try Biotech Health in Petersfield, particularly a nutritionist called Anne Smitten. I think this was the wisest money I have spent on my way to recovery.

Food intolerance and vitamin/mineral screening showed I could eat only fruit, vegetables, some grains and nuts. My body could not absorb any vitamins in tablet form. I had been taking just such tablets from the health store. Her tests showed that by doing this I was simply loading myself with even more toxins and making my liver work harder to digest all of it.

I went home with a clear plan for the next six months:

1. Detox
2. Diet
3. Nutrition
4. Coffee Enemas

As Anne likes to say, 'One thing at a time. We have to be patient with you. When you get cancer, it means you have probably been doing something wrong for a long period of 3–5 years minimum, so to fix it will take time as well. We have to get your body to change part of its chemistry'.

I also had a hair analysis at the Wellbeing Clinic that showed a very high mercury level in my body. So I found a holistic dentist to remove my amalgam fillings, which can leak heavy metals into the body and overstretch the immune system. I had a special heavy metal detox programme after the fillings were removed.

In summer 2003, as part of my vacation, I visited the clinic in Moscow where photodynamic therapy (PDT) was created. They use what they call a photosensitise — a solution that is taken orally, and when combined with laser light, kills tumours. There are no cumulative toxic effects with PDT as with radiation and chemotherapy, so the procedure can be repeated several times if needed. The Dove Clinic for Integrated Medicine offers this in the UK.

Dr Kenyon from the clinic recommended C-Statin for me. This is made from bindweed. The theory is that this contains inhibitors which stop the body from growing new blood vessels to supply tumours, which then cannot grow. Whilst I was in Russia, I was introduced to Irina Filipova, Professor of Fungotherapy (mushrooms). She tailor-made a plan for me, which included five types of mushrooms and some herbs. I have been taking this for one year now and have a great belief in it.

As I am in early menopause following my hysterectomy and have all the usual symptoms, I looked for a way to regulate my hot flushes and have found acupuncture to be of great assistance. My CA-125 is stable, within the normal range. I am enjoying life and every day is a special gift for me.

I would like to thank all the people who helped me through this very difficult time, especially my husband and all of the staff at the C&W, particularly Mr J Richard Smith and Dr M Bower.

Recollections of Galina Dean's husband, John

Ovarian Cancer: A Husband's Experience

Today is the fourth anniversary of the day on which I met my wife, Galina ('Gala'). In late summer 2002, without any warning, she was diagnosed with Stage IV ovarian cancer at the age of 38. In this circumstance, one is immediately aware that the role of the husband is that of a supporting player in a drama where nature is in control.

We experienced both extremes of the NHS during the first three months. The worst — anger and frustration at our GP's refusal to take my wife's symptoms seriously, seemingly more concerned about the use of NHS resources in requesting any tests which would have revealed the problem 5–6 weeks before it was finally discovered. This was in light of the fact that Gala had an abdominal scar having had an ovary removed with a benign cyst 20 years earlier. The best — first class care and attention at the hands of the oncology team under Dr Mark Bower at Chelsea and Westminster Hospital and the surgical team under Mr J Richard Smith.

We will never know whether the delay has affected Gala's probability of survival. However, it is clear that without the help of the people at Chelsea & Westminster, she would not be alive today!

Whilst being aware that Gala's body has to fight this problem, I have tried in my small way to make it a shared problem. I believe that all husbands can make a difference in these circumstances. Whether or not it is admitted, anyone who is diagnosed with cancer is scared of dying and needs reassurance that there is always a chance of survival.

One should be aware of the statistics, but one should never accept that the worst outcome is inevitable. I tried, wherever possible, to attend all meetings with Gala and to always drive her to the hospital and to which ever clinic she was attending. We went to the Paracelsus Klinic in Switzerland together and I met with all of her doctors. I believe that it is important to try to retain a measure of control over one's own destiny. For example, Gala knew that she would lose her long hair (a prized asset!) and so after the first treatment, we found an understanding hairdresser, who gave her a No. 1 cut and also advised on the purchase of a wig.

My advice is — do not be afraid to spend money on a good wig, even at the expense of some other seemingly necessary items. Nothing is more important at this time than maintaining self-confidence and self-esteem. In Gala's case although she was extremely upset to lose her hair, she controlled the moment of loss herself. She also consoled herself with the knowledge that it was virtually certain to grow back stronger than ever.

I believe that the key is an open mind, a positive attitude and a determination to explore all avenues for treatment, both within traditional and non-traditional medicine. It seems to me that although brutal and toxic, chemotherapy and surgery are necessary evils. Galina has met a number of people who have only been prepared to undertake non-traditional solutions, but in my opinion, one reduces the probability for survival if traditional medical treatment is ignored.

I can only share with you our experiences and cannot say that this will work for everyone, but (fingers crossed) it is working for Gala. Her CA-125 (tumour marker) numbers have gone from 2,700 before chemo to 7 as of today, and are stable around this figure (normal range 0–23).

Anything that increases belief in survival has to be a good thing. It may be that some of the things that we have tried for Gala have simply increased her belief in her own survival rather than being effective in their own right. I do not think that this is the case, but even if it is, I would still go ahead with them. I am generally a sceptical person and I do not understand some of the treatments that she has received, but I have seen the results with my own eyes.

After a course of chemotherapy, one is faced with the fact that for a period, no further treatments of this type can be undertaken for a long period. We therefore concentrated on three areas in looking for alternatives. We wanted to detoxify her body after the effects of the chemotherapy and also get rid of any heavy metals, which could be inhibiting her immune system. We then concentrated on treatments that would generally boost her immune system. One of the first revelations for me was the fact that everyone produces cancerous cells continuously and one's immune system normally kills them.

Finally, we tried to find a treatment that would kill cancer cells without the toxic effects of traditional chemotherapy. Gala has listed all the treatments that she has found to be useful. This may not be a comprehensive list and I would encourage everyone to explore all avenues to discover more diverse remedies. We could not find such a list when we started and it is entirely due to Gala's determination that we have covered the treatments mentioned.

In conclusion, this experience has brought us closer together. We believe in the strategy that we have evolved for Gala and are grateful for each day. She is in remission and her tests are within the normal range. It is still early days and we cannot take anything for granted.

Commentary by Richard Smith

Originally, I had not intended to make any comment upon the pieces kindly written above. However, having read them and digested them, I have to say I find each deeply moving and all in different ways. It is purely by chance that all three patients should have adopted different strategies for coping with and handling their disease. It is important to say that there were no other pieces solicited which have subsequently been 'spiked' (edited out) because they did not happen to suit. I am not able to comment upon many of the complementary therapies that Galina has described. Her piece does remind me of Michael Gerin-Tosh's very moving and important book, *Living Proof — A Medical Mutiny* (see recommended reading).

I do however believe that Galina, while accessing a range of complementary therapies, has also rightly used the orthodox ones as well. John Diamond, in his book *Snakedance*, takes the opposite approach to Gearin-Tosh, namely dismissing most complimentary therapies. As stated on many occasions in this book, I personally believe that different strategies suit different patients and a combination of orthodox and complementary therapies are advantageous; the three pieces here amply demonstrate this.

Finally, I know that Galina and her husband feel very aggrieved by their GP and the failure to make an earlier diagnosis. This is very understandable. I believe I should say, however, that most patients with advanced ovarian cancer have usually taken some time to get diagnosed. This is not just down to incompetence, but to the very real difficulty of making the diagnosis. The ovaries are not visible without sophisticated scanning, and the symptoms cancer on the ovary produces are often vague and difficult to interpret. This gives GPs and, for that matter, gynaecologists difficulties in making the diagnosis. The vexed subject of screening is covered on pages 78–81 which further elaborates on this difficult subject. I would, however, entirely concur with Galina that if you have persistent symptoms, to go back and let your doctor know.

We now return to examples of other patients.

Patient 3

A 60-year-old woman comes into the ward complaining of being unable to control urination. In fact, she is permanently passing urine through her vagina. She has had treatment for an advanced cancer of the cervix three years earlier with radiotherapy and chemotherapy. All had gone well (**Cusp B**) until a few weeks ago when the urinary problems had started. She had been examined in the clinic and unfortunately, her tumour had returned and had created a hole between her bladder and vagina. Her kidneys are also failing, so she is in **Cusp C**; in other words, she is no longer curable. She is unsuitable for surgery, further chemotherapy or radiotherapy. She was told these facts and that she had recurrent incurable cancer.

She said she had already guessed this and she was very angry. She was then asked the vital question for **Cusp C**, which is: 'I am very sorry to be giving you this news, but is it that you are going to die in the next few weeks or months that is making you angry or is there something else which is troubling you?' It could be pain, constipation, etc. To this question, the woman replied that she accepted the inevitability of impending death but, much worse, she had been told by someone else that nothing else could be done for her. She was asked, 'I know that in terms of curing you, none of us can help you, but what is your biggest problem right now?' To this, she replied that her biggest problem now was her incontinence and the fact that she smelt of urine permanently. Because of this she could not go out, could not visit friends or be visited. She was asked what other problems she was having to which she replied 'none'! At this point, it was possible to say to her that although there was no gynaecological treatment, there was a colleague downstairs who is an interventional radiologist, a specialist in using X-rays to visualise the body, who could insert a tube into each kidney, to drain urine away, thus bypassing the hole in her bladder and rendering her dry and smell-free! (See Figure 3.6.)

The patient went home the following day, and returned two months later in a terminal condition (**Cusp D**). On return, she said she had had a great two months, seen her friends, been to restaurants, pubs, etc. In this woman's case, death came within 24 hours and was peaceful.

The fourth cusp lasts from hours to days and all interventions are only designed to ease the passing. Patients, in general, need no telling that this is where they have arrived, although their relatives may need help in arriving at this place. Care is focused on emotional support rather than medical intervention and, frequently, most of the patient's medicines can be stopped apart from pain relief. The death of a patient whose physical symptoms are well controlled and who is spiritually calm is an achievable goal to which all are entitled.

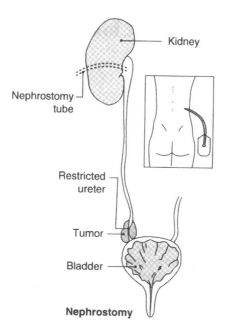

Nephrostomy

Figure 3.6   Nephrostomy.

Chapter 4

General Concepts of Surgical Management

The fact that you are reading this book is almost certainly because you or a relative have been diagnosed as having cancer. The process by which that diagnosis was made will, I know, have caused you great distress and seemed to have taken ages. For the majority of you, hopefully, it will have taken no more than a few weeks, but those few weeks will have been psychologically and/or physically painful and stressful. You will almost certainly have gone to your GP, perhaps with a swelling in your tummy or some irregularity of bleeding or perhaps with pain. Your GP will have examined you, performed tests and referred you either to a general gynaecologist or to some form of rapid assessment clinic or perhaps directly to a gynaecological cancer specialist. A gynaecological cancer specialist will be a highly trained surgeon who will have specially trained in the area and will be somebody who you can feel certain is up to date in modern management of gynaecological cancer, who understands the different types of treatment and will work within a large team of individuals. These teams meet at what are called multi-disciplinary team (MDT) meetings on a regular (weekly or fortnightly) basis. At these meetings there are usually a minimum of two or more surgeons, a radiotherapist, one or more medical oncologists who prescribe chemotherapy, a radiologist who takes and reads ultrasound scans, X-rays, computerised tomography (CT), positron emission tomography (PET)-CT, and magnetic resonance imaging (MRI) scans, specialist oncology nurses and a pathologist. All of these consultants may well have junior members in their respective teams who will also attend these meetings and who you may see during your care. These meetings ensure that the treatment that you are offered is the optimal treatment and so that no one group (e.g. the surgeon or the radiotherapist) can steer you into the wrong therapy.

What follows relates to referrals to the gynaecologic oncologist when referrals are made for a cancer. This does not include patients with abnormal smears who are sent for colposcopy. If you are in this category, please go the section on colposcopy on pages 58–61.

When you come to the clinic, you may initially have your history taken; in other words, you will be asked about your medical 'story' to date. This may be done by a medical student or a junior doctor in the first instance. Medical students take five years in training and your 'junior doctor' in the UK may be qualified from one week to ten years; i.e. some are not very 'junior'! In the USA, the range is one week to seven years. It is important to let you know of the hierarchy. In the UK, there are Foundation Year (FY) doctors, which entails working in multiple specialities in the first two years following qualifying. This is followed by Speciality Training (ST) (years 1–7), the last two years of which includes Subspeciality Training (years 6–7), where trainees focus on a specific area within the speciality, such as gynaecology oncology. The old Senior Registrar is now an ST 6-7. The subspecialist trainee is, in other words, very senior, 10–12 years post qualification. One of the authors (JRS) conducted an informal survey of patients in clinic to see how they perceived the titles and seniority and the term subspecialist trainee is almost universally misunderstood to be somebody junior rather than senior. In the USA, there are Residents (years 1–4), Chief Residents (year 5), and subspecialist fellows (years 6–8).

After the history, you will be examined. This usually involves having both your tummy examined and a pelvic examination. This should not be painful but may occasionally be uncomfortable. Investigations are then ordered, including blood tests, usually for kidney function (urea and electrolytes) a full blood count to check for anaemia, liver function tests and a blood test called tumour markers. These tests tend to rise with cancers, although certain benign conditions can cause a rise as well. Scans and X-rays will be ordered for you. These may be by ultrasound, CT, MRI or PET.

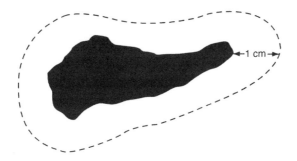

Figure 4.1   Tumour being removed with a minimum of a 1 cm clear margin around it.

None of these tests are painful. All these tests are designed to help determine whether the tumour is benign or cancerous/malignant. If there is a cancer, they will help to show if it has spread or not; this is called 'radiological staging'. This will all be explained to you. Many people require to go on to have surgery and all the appropriate operations are described in the relevant chapter for each cancer type. Many cancers are then 'restaged' on the basis of the surgical findings and results of the analyses performed on the samples obtained (histopathology and cytopathology).

The general principle of how surgery works remains the same for all cancers. It is to remove an abnormal lump preferably with a 1-cm area of normal tissue around it (see Figure 4.1). This is then analysed in the pathology laboratory to determine whether it is cancerous and if it is, whether it has been completely removed, thus avoiding the need for further treatment, while achieving a cure.

In summary, whenever one has surgery for a suspected cancer, there are three outcomes: firstly, the problem proves to be benign and the surgery is likely to be the solution to the problem; secondly, it is cancerous but completely excised and the problem solved; or thirdly, it is cancerous and perhaps not completely excised and further therapy will be required.

Chapter 5

Sex, Cancer and Surgery

When a woman develops cancer in her genital tract, be it on the vulva (the outside of the vagina), the vagina itself, the cervix, uterus, tubes or ovaries, it is often the presumption that it is in some way related to sex. Often people harbour feelings of guilt as to whether they have done something wrong in the past that is now coming back to them in the form of a cancer. This impression has been further fostered by much of the tabloid press, where there regularly appear articles, suggesting that such and such cancer is because of 'promiscuity'. The definition of 'promiscuity', that medical students are given, is the patient having had one more partner than their doctor! It is really a totally meaningless term. One person's promiscuity is another person's normality. Having said all of this, it is true that endometrial cancer is associated with never having been sexually active and not having had children.

It is also true that taking the oral contraceptive pill for five years reduces your chances of ovarian cancer by 40% and if you take it for ten years, your chance goes down by 70%. This does presuppose that you do not have breaks. It is very unfortunate that currently in the 'ether', many young women believe they should 'detox' themselves of the 'pill' regularly. This practice is wrong, maximises the risks and reduces the benefits.

It is also true that using condoms offers some protection from human papilloma virus infection (HPV) and this virus is implicated in causing cervical cancer. Having said this, they do not offer much protection and probably up to 85% of all men and women at some time in their lives will have HPV, irrespective of the number of partners, but an incredibly low percentage of these will ever go on to develop cervical cancer itself. In discordant couples, where one has HPV and the other does not at the start of their relationship, if no condoms are used, there is a 100% transmission of HPV within six episodes of sex. If condoms are used, there is a 100% transmission rate after 12 episodes of sex. If you look at the cervical cancer chapter (Chapter 6), you will see that there is much talk about cervical intra-epithelial neoplasia (CIN), which is the cell change that takes place before women get cervical cancer. It has been, to my mind, extremely unfortunate that CIN, which should be stated by using the initials C, I, N has occasionally been referred to as 'sin'. It is obvious that anybody hearing a doctor talk about 'sin' would immediately think that this must be related to something which they have done wrong! This is really just not the way it is!

Many women also worry as to what effect the treatment of their cancer will have upon sexual function. It is true to say that for the majority of gynaecological cancers, you will be able to resume a normal sexual life afterwards.

Sex is a complicated mixture of the psychological and the physical. Whenever something goes wrong with the reproductive organs, this is likely to have some psychological effect at least in the first instance. Depending upon which part of the organs are affected, this may affect sexual function afterwards and in addition, it obviously does depend upon which operation you have as to what effect this may have. For this reason I have included a section on sexual aspects of treatments, etc. in each of the chapters related to that particular cancer.

Overall, it is thought that in terms of orgasm, there are four types of women: women who do not achieve orgasm, women who achieve orgasm through stimulation of the clitoris and external genitalia, women who achieve orgasm by deep penetration, and the fourth group, namely, those women who achieve orgasm by both routes. The famous 'G' spot is a much disputed entity and if it exists, it perhaps exists occasionally in the cervix or, more commonly, related to the plexus of nerves in the front wall of the vagina, high up near the base of the bladder. These considerations are important, since for the majority of people having surgery for gynaecological cancer this tends to involve either removal of an ovary or both ovaries, neither of which have any direct effect on sexual function, except via hormones, and they may need HRT. Removal of the uterus will probably also have no effect on sexual function. Removal of the cervix may affect deep orgasmic function, but probably doesn't in the majority of woman. The evidence is that the majority of women following hysterectomy have an improved sex life and that removal of the cervix makes no difference to that pleasure. It is unusual for gynaecological surgery to involve the vagina itself, unless there is a tumour that has spread onto the vagina.

Finally, for the small number of women where the vulva is affected, attempts, particularly in young women, are made to preserve as much vulval tissue as is possible, again with a view to preserving sexual function. Even women who have had a vulvectomy may still be capable of achieving orgasm, via the deep vaginal stimulation route. There is no doubting that radiotherapy to the pelvis greatly reduces the elasticity of pelvic organs and this can have a deleterious effect on sex. In addition, it can be associated with dryness, although there are good vaginal lubricants available to alleviate dryness. It is terribly important that if you are having sexual problems that you bring this up with your gynaecological oncologist or with the specialist nurse, since there are usually things that can be done to help matters. There is a natural reticence on the part of many doctors/ nurses to directly ask about this area and a natural reticence on the part of the patients to not ask either.

Section II
Information on
Specific Cancers

Chapter 6

Cervical Cancer and Pre-Cancer (Cervical Intra-Epithelial Neoplasia (CIN)/Squamous Intra-Epithelial Lesion (SIL))

General Facts

No one knows exactly how common cervical cancer is. The 'incidence' or rate varies in different parts of the world and in different parts of each country. The disease is more common in cities and less common in rural areas. It tends to be commoner in populations with lower socio-economic status, although higher economic status is no bar to developing the disease.

Cervical cancer is known to be associated with smoking because smoking has a direct effect on local immune cells in the cervix. It is also known to be associated with a poor immune system, for example, after having had an organ transplant and needing immunosuppressive drug treatment or as a result of HIV infection. It is very important to say that the vast majority of women who have CIN do not have HIV or, for that matter, have had an organ transplant. In addition, women with an abnormal smear have only the slightest increased risk of having HIV. Although a positive HIV test is very unlikely, you may be offered this test. This is part of a wider drive to increase HIV testing across the whole population.

Most women when they have an abnormal smear test believe that they have cervical cancer. This is almost always untrue. Long before developing

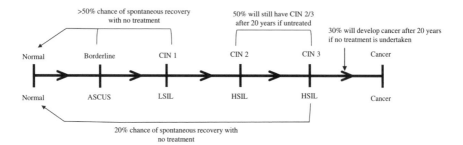

Figure 6.1   The sliding scale from normal to cervical cancer. CIN = cervical intra-epithe-lial neoplasia, ASCUS = abnormal smear of uncertain clinical significance, LSIL = low grade squamous intra-epithelial lesion, HSIL = high grade intra-epithelial lesion.

cervical cancer, cell changes take place in the cervix and these are graded into CIN 1/LSIL, 2 and 3/HSIL. CIN is the UK, European term and stands for cervical intra-epithelial cancer; SIL is the USA terminology and stands for squamous intra-epithelial lesion (i.e. NOT cancer but PRE-cancer). Cancers can spread distantly, but CIN/SIL cannot. The dual classification and the sliding scale from normal to cervical cancer are shown in Figure 6.1.

From here, the text will stick to the UK classification for ease of reading.

Even before development of CIN 1, smears become borderline first. As can be seen from the diagram, you can draw arrows showing that some women's smears go from normal to borderline and then from borderline to CIN 1, progressing to CIN 2, and finally to CIN 3. **If you had a CIN 3 diagnosis (and had no treatment) and did nothing about it, you would have a 30% chance that by the time 20 years had gone by, you would have developed cervical cancer.** Conversely, you would have a 20% chance that your smear would have gone back to normal on its own and a 50% chance that the smear would remain as CIN 3. CIN 1, 2 and 3 all cause no symptoms; they cause no pain, no bleeding and no discharge and, in fact, in themselves are not a problem. The problem is that they may develop into cervical cancer if left untreated. The lesser condition of CIN 1 has a higher chance of returning to normal with an approximately 50% chance of returning to normal within 6–12 months of diagnosis. This is the reason why you may have been told that you have an abnormal smear but the only action being taken is to repeat the smear a few months later. This particularly applies to borderline smears, again where there is a good chance of resolution (50–60%) happening without you requiring any treatment at all. The factors that primarily make some women's smears go from normal through to CIN 3, and others not, tend to be either heavy smoking or, more commonly, the acquisition of a type of virus called HPV. HPV stands for human papilloma virus. There are many types of HPV, some of which cause warts on the genitals (HPV 6+11); other types cause warts on the fingers. The types of HPV that cause CIN (HPV 16, 18, 31, 33, 35, 39, 45, 51, 52, 56, 58, 59, and 68) do not, however, cause warts. This can often lead to confusion since colloquially HPV is often known as the 'wart virus'; the confusion being that the types of HPV that cause CIN do **not** cause warts. In addition, HPV 16 causes 50% of all high grade lesions (CIN 2, 3), HPV 18 causes 20%, and HPV 31 and 33 a further 15%. In other words, 85% of high grade lesions are caused by just four of the HPV types. This is why the mRNA test described below concentrates on these tests.

To create further difficulties in this part of the explanation, when you have a standard smear test taken, there may be cells seen which are 'suggestive of HPV'. This does not mean that you actually have HPV and it is not possible from looking at these cells to see which type of HPV is present, or even if it is HPV and not some other virus. Epstein Barr virus, which causes glandular fever, can cause this type of cell change, but does **not** cause CIN. The only way to do this is by direct testing for the virus. This direct test is now commonly available, although not universally. Where the test is available, there may be two tests: DNA and mRNA.

With the DNA test, one of the available tests (DYGENE, a USA developed test) tells you if any of the HPV types mentioned above are positive; it does not say which one or indeed if more than one is positive. The alternate HPV DNA test tells you which of the different types is positive. If you are positive for HPV 16, 18, 31, 33, or 45, then the Norchip proofer mRNA test can automatically be performed. If the mRNA is positive, then it is likely that progression will take place unless there is treatment and, therefore, treatment will usually be offered. If the DNA is positive, but the mRNA is negative, it is likely that things will return to normal without treatment. In clinics where DNA testing alone is available, persistence of a positive DNA test will lead to treatment.

Table 6.1   Action in the event of cervical smear result.

RESULT	ACTION
Normal	Repeat as per national policy
Inflammatory/ borderline (in the USA = ASCUS)	Screen for sexually transmitted infections (STIs). Repeat at 6 months, utilise HPV testing. If HPV negative, return to standard recall.
Suggestive of CIN 1 (in the USA = LSIL)	Colposcopy, repeat at 6 months, utilise HPV testing. If HPV negative, return to standard recall.
Suggestive of CIN 2 (in the USA = HSIL)	Refer for colposcopy
Suggestive of CIN 3 (in the USA = HSIL)	Refer for colposcopy
Suggestive of invasion (cancer) (very unusual result)	Refer for colposcopy, urgent

For those clinics that have access to the HPV testing kit, the results are used as a method of determining whether to treat CIN 1 or not. If there is a very small area of CIN 2, then the HPV test may be used to determine whether to treat or not. If the area of CIN 2 is large, it is always treated. CIN 3 is always treated and I will discuss the treatment shortly. CIN 1 is only treated if it is persistent and/or in the presence of a positive HPV test (if this test is available). If this test is not available, then CIN 1 is only usually treated if it is present on two occasions at least six months apart. The actions taken, depending upon the result, are shown in the following table.

There is currently a new screening process being developed whereby HPV will be tested for first: if negative, no smear (cytology) is required; if positive, a smear is performed; if abnormal CIN 1 or greater, the patient is referred for colposcopy. If borderline repeat both tests at six months and if still HPV positive and borderline, refer for colposcopy.

Explanation as to How CIN Arises

The area of the cervix (neck of the womb) that has the potential to develop CIN is called the transformation zone and it is formed after puberty. Figure 6.2 shows what happens at puberty. The inside of the cervix has

Pre-puberty	'Normal' cervix	Cervical ectopy	Postmenopausal cervix

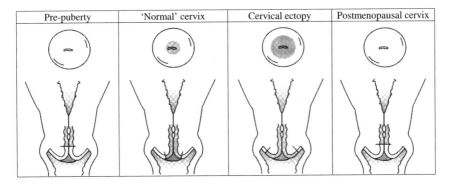

Figure 6.2 Cervical changes over a reproductive lifetime.

fleshy cells called columnar cells and on the outside, it has squamous cells. Squamous cells are tough cells. At puberty, under the influence of the hormones which are released in all women, the cervix undergoes a process of eversion (out turning). This means that the fleshy columnar cells appear out on the surface. The vagina is then colonised with bacteria; these bacteria are normal to have in the vagina. In fact, to not have them is positively harmful; they are called lactobacilli. These lactobacilli are the same lactobacilli found in live yoghurt, which are often used to prevent thrush. They cause the acidity in the vagina to increase. This, however, causes the fleshy columnar cells to change their nature and become tougher and to change into the squamous cells (i.e. to transform). The area where this change takes place is the area that has the capacity to develop CIN. This area is called the transformation zone and, as you can see from the picture, the transformation zone can vary from being on the outside of the cervix to the inside of the cervix. These are all just different variations of normal. They do, however, slightly alter the treatment depending on their position.

It is the fact that a pre-cancerous condition exists in the cervix — in other words, the cell change that takes place many years before actual cancer — which makes it suitable for screening with smears. It is vitally important to realise that CIN is NOT cancer. Cancer means that a lesion has the capacity to metastasise; in other words, to spread through the body. CIN has no such capacity. We also know that CIN 1 never directly becomes cervical cancer; it always becomes CIN 2–3 before becoming cervical cancer.

It is these facts that make it safe to observe CIN 1 and make the relatively simple treatment offered for CIN 2 and 3 appropriate, giving a very high success rate in preventing women from developing cervical cancer.

One of the things that often causes confusion is how often smears are undertaken and Table 6.2 shows the detection rates of CIN for cervical smears being taken at varying intervals. As you can see, the current National Health Service (NHS) guideline is three yearly, which delivers a 'hit rate' of 89%. As described above, the UK screening is about to change radically by relying on HPV testing. Most other countries operate on the basis of an annual screening test, but this only gives a 4.5% gain in detection rate, while effectively doubling the cost of the entire programme. It is, therefore, in terms of running a programme effectively, most important to screen all of the people regularly, rather than some of the people a lot!

There is an irony, since the smear programme in the UK has had a lot of bad publicity over the years with regards to unreliability, and much unfavourable press when smears are occasionally missed. The irony is that the smear programme is undoubtedly one of the 'jewels in the crown' of the UK's NHS and in terms of the efficiency of the programme's purpose, namely to reduce the incidence of invasive cancer within a specified population, it is one of the most successful programmes in the world. Unfortunately, all medical tests have a false positive and a false negative rate; in other words, they are reported as abnormal when there is no problem, or they are reported as normal when in fact there is a problem. It is for this reason that, over time, the more smears one has, the better it is and

Table 6.2 Detection rates for cervical screening[*] at varying screening intervals (%).

Screening Interval	%
10-yearly	64
5-yearly	84
3-yearly	89
Annually	93.5

[*]Sexually active woman are screened between the ages of 20 and 69 years.

the more accurate it is. The long time that CIN takes to develop into invasive cancer also makes it very suitable for screening purposes. The false negative rate of smears, namely when they are reported as normal when in fact they are abnormal, comes down to laboratory error or down to error in taking the smear. It is possible to take the smear from not quite the right area, although this happens rarely.

The Way the Smear is Taken

For those of you who have had smears taken for more than ten years, you may remember that the doctor used a wooden spatula and a device that looked like a little brush. The sample was put on a glass slide. This method of doing smears has been entirely superseded by liquid cytology: a Thin prep smear® (Registered trade name) is used, which utilises a device called the 'broom'. This device has the advantage that one can also directly test for HPV from the same sample and run a screen for other infections. It also means smears can be taken when you are on your period unless the bleeding is heavy. This is because the sample is centrifuged (i.e. spun) and the red blood cells can be removed leaving the cervical cells that need to be examined. It is very important if you have bleeding between your periods and/or after sex that the doctor examines you even if you are bleeding. Most women are naturally reticent to be examined when they are bleeding. While this is completely understandable, it is very important that the cervix is visualised to exclude polyps and more importantly, but rarely, cervical cancer.

When you have a smear test, it is either reported as normal or abnormal and the standard approach has already been shown in Table 6.1 In the event of an inflammatory smear, a screen for infection is undertaken. This screen tests routinely for Chlamydia, gonorrhoea, Group B streptococcus, trichomonas, candida and bacterial vaginosis. It is important to say that the Group B streptococcus and bacterial vaginosis are not sexually transmitted. Candida can be, but you can have candida and be a nun! Chlamydia is a sexually transmitted agent, but is not a venereal disease (i.e. the discovery of it does not mean that you or your partner have been unfaithful to each other). The same does not apply to gonorrhoea, which is a statutory venereal disease; in other words, it is suggestive of either you or your partner having had another partner. Having said this, there are certain tests for gonorrhoea that are used for rapid testing and these can be positive when you don't actually have gonorrhoea. This is called a false positive and occurs because of a cross-reaction of the test with non-sexually transmitted throat bacteria. It is important to point out that HPV is extremely common. Approximately up to 85% of all men and women will have HPV at some point in their lives and while it is a marker of sexual activity, it is in no way a venereal disease. One of the reasons it is so common is its ease of transmission. In a discordant couple, where one partner has an infection and the other does not, with HPV, there is 100% transmission within six episodes of sex if no condoms have been used. With condoms, if they have twelve episodes of sex, it gives 100% transmission. This is in contrast to HIV, where to get 100% transmission, you would need over a thousand episodes of sexual intercourse.

It should also be remembered that if >50% of the population have something, then it cannot be regarded as abnormal to have it — in fact it's normal to have it. Of the 85% who have HPV, the vast majority don't ever get a problem from it, with only 5 to 10% getting an abnormal smear. Although it does not seem particularly fair, men usually get no problem from HPV and we don't test or treat the male partner nor do we treat the woman for HPV unless it is the variety that causes warts. These are treated because of their unsightly nature. Also, remember that the type of HPV that causes warts (HPV 6+11) does not cause CIN. Most women with HPV will clear it themselves within an 18-month period. One exception to this may be women who smoke heavily because of smoking's effect on the immune cells, which inhibits the ability to naturally clear the virus. There is some data to suggest that a heavy smoker who quits smoking may have a better chance of her smear returning to normal without treatment. If you have an abnormal smear, you will be sent for a colposcopy.

Colposcopy

This word is derived from *colpos*, which is Greek for 'vagina', and *scopy*, 'to look', and in the same way as your doctor or practice nurse took the smear by looking at your cervix with the naked eye; the only difference is that a colposcopist (i.e., a gynaecologist performing the colposcopy) will look at your cervix through the same type of speculum (viewing instrument), but this time looking down a binocular microscope (see Figure 6.3

for further details). This is not a painful examination, but the binocular microscope allows 4–20 times normal magnification. When you go to the colposcopy clinic, you can expect the gynaecologist to take a history from you and then to explain to you that they will probably repeat your smear. They will explain that smears are designed to detect pre-cancer and not cancer. Assuming that your doctor/nurse who originally took your smear has thought that your cervix looked normal, then the chances of you having a cancer are incredibly low. Cancers are almost always seen by directly looking at the cervix and there is no requirement for a colposcope/microscope. CIN is a microscopic condition; in other words, it is not visible with the naked eye, only with a microscope. The doctor will then give you a similar explanation to the one given in the previous pages with respect to CIN. You will then be taken through to another room where you will be placed on a couch and the examination will be undertaken. Dyes are placed on the cervix. The first dye is usually merely saline (salt water), which is designed to clean the cervix. This will then be followed by a very dilute solution of acetic acid (vinegar). This does not cause stinging or pain. The final dye placed may be iodine (unless you are allergic to iodine). Occasionally, this can cause slight discomfort. If it does, washing with saline (salt water) gives immediate relief. Depending on what is seen, biopsies (small samples) may be taken from the cervix. The doctor may suggest that you cough, which makes the cervix bounce down and makes it easier to get the sample. It also usually has the advantage that you don't feel the sample being taken at all, which nobody believes until after they have had the sample taken. Occasionally a slight 'nip' is felt at the time of sampling. This sample will then be sent for analysis along with the repeat smear test if this has been done, and the colposcopic findings to allow a judgement to be made. The act of taking the biopsy may also stimulate your cervix to make an immune response, which may help you to clear HPV and CIN 1 without treatment.

In the past, many gynaecologists used to do 'see and treat'. This meant that if upon colposcopy you had CIN, they would immediately treat you. This was justifiable particularly in areas where many of the patients would default on their clinic appointments. However, in the last few years, data has appeared that shows that although the risks of treatment are low, there is a slight risk of premature labour and mid-trimester (between 12 and 24 weeks)

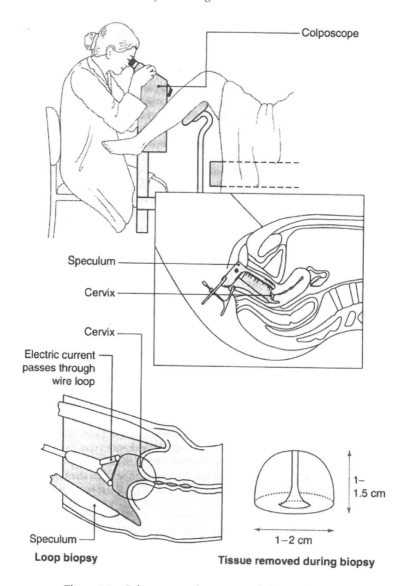

Figure 6.3   Colposcopy and treatment of abnormal smear.

- Colposcopy is carried out if the smear test shows up abnormalities in the cervical cells. A colposcope is a microscope that magnifies the cervix.
- Colposcopy is a painless, outpatient procedure. You will be asked to lie on your back with your legs in supports.
- A plastic or metal instrument called a speculum is inserted into the vagina to hold the walls of the vagina apart. The speculum is similar to that used for a smear.

◄──

Figure 6.3 *(Continue on facing page)*

- Dilute acetic acid, and possibly iodine, will be painted onto your cervix to show up any abnormalities. Small samples of tissue, called biopsies, may be taken from the cervix and sent to the laboratory for analysis. These procedures do not hurt, but may be a bit uncomfortable.
- During colposcopy, abnormal cervical cells can be removed or destroyed in a number of ways. The most common is called loop biopsy or LLETZ. A local anaesthetic is injected to numb your cervix. This is not painful, but may be uncomfortable. A small piece of tissue containing the abnormal cells is then removed using an electrical current; the sample removed is about the size of a marble. Other methods involve heating or freezing the area with the abnormal cells, or removing or destroying it using a laser.
- You are likely to have discharge and abnormal bleeding for a few weeks after treatment. If the bleeding is heavy or if the discharge becomes offensive, consult your doctor.

miscarriage. In addition, we know many women with CIN 1 will spontaneously revert to normal and even a few women with CIN 2 will do this. For these reasons, most of the time now, your doctor will want to get all your results together at a later date and then treat you if appropriate.

Prevention: HPV Vaccination

In the last few years, most developed countries have introduced vaccination to prevent HPV infection. There are two vaccines available: one that protects against HPV 16 and 18, and another that protects against 16, 18, 6 and 11. The former two cause 70% of cases of CIN; however, it now seems there is an added benefit in protecting against HPV 31 and 33, so perhaps 80% of cases will be prevented. It is most effective if given prior to starting sexual activity, hence most programmes vaccinate girls at school at approximately 12 years of age. The vaccine is entirely safe with a tiny number of girls being allergic and unable to finish the course of three shots spread over 6–12 months. It is very important that girls know they will still need to have smears even if they have had the vaccine. The vaccines are to prevent infection and have no role in treating somebody who already has HPV 16 or 18. There is, however, some new data suggesting that even after treatment of CIN, there may be some benefit of vaccination in future prevention of HPV infection. The vaccine is licensed up until aged 50 years. The authors have both seen women in their forties who, following divorce and before looking to form a new relationship, have requested and been given the vaccination.

Treatment of Abnormalities

In the past, up until 20–25 years ago, it used to be that treatments had to be dealt with as an inpatient under general anaesthetic. These were done using a knife to remove an area from the cervix. Over the last 20–25 years, a number of treatments have become available for outpatient use. The first of these was freezing therapy (cryotherapy) and this is still sometimes used for treatment of CIN 1. In persistently borderline smears, it has about an 80% chance of working, is simple to use and pain-free, except for some slight occasional period-like cramping pain. It does not require any local anaesthetic.

The next treatment that became available was laser treatment. Most people have now moved away from using laser treatment, partly because it takes quite some time to undertake the treatment, particularly if one wishes to produce a sample to send to the pathology department. Most clinics now use a large loop excision of the transformation zone (LLETZ loop) (as shown in Figure 6.4). Needle excision can also be undertaken (NETZ). Both of these allow removal of an ellipse of tissue as shown in the diagram,

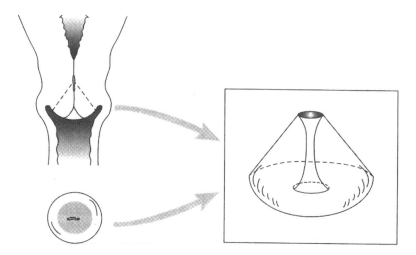

Figure 6.4   Local treatment of the transformation zone.

which allows both removal of the abnormal area plus further investigation of the abnormal area, all effectively in one episode. In a further small number of people who have pre-cancerous changes on the vagina, vaginal intra-epithelial neoplasia (VAIN), the laser or more recently, PlasmaJet®, is used.

A very small number of women will be found, either on examination by their GP or on examination in the colposcopy clinic, to have a cervical cancer (cervical carcinoma). This is a different phenomenon from CIN. As stated above, CIN is the microscopic change that precedes cancer, usually by many years. Usually a person with cervical cancer is referred to the colposcopy clinic because the doctor taking the smear recognises that the cervix has appeared very abnormal and makes an immediate referral. Occasionally the referral may be because the smear is suggestive of malignancy. Sometimes the LLETZ loop sample may show a cancer that was previously unsuspected — this is very uncommon. The other method by which women sometimes come to see the gynaecologist is because they have had problems (e.g. bleeding between periods or bleeding after sex) and are seen and the doctor or nurse recognises a cancer. With an effective screening programme, this has become a much rarer way of people being diagnosed.

Cervical Cancer

Figure 6.5 provides an overview on cervical cancer.

Whenever a cancer is diagnosed, it is 'staged'. This refers to whether it has spread or not. When a cancer is 'named', it is always 'named' after where it has started (e.g. lung cancer has arisen in the lung). Sometimes, it is not clear where the cancer has started; this is called an 'unknown primary'. Thus, cancer in the cervix starts in the cervix and as it spreads, it can move slowly through the cervix and then onto the vagina or out to the side of the cervix. In addition, it can also spread into the lymph nodes. Occasionally it can spread further towards the bladder or bowel. It very rarely spreads through the bloodstream. Because it very rarely spreads through the bloodstream, it is a type of cancer that has a relatively high cure rate and the cure is usually obtained by therapies that concentrate on the pelvic area. The first investigations once a diagnosis of cancer is suspected are to determine whether the cancer has spread or not. These incorporate blood tests, chest X-ray and MRI scanning of the pelvis and the lymph nodes within the

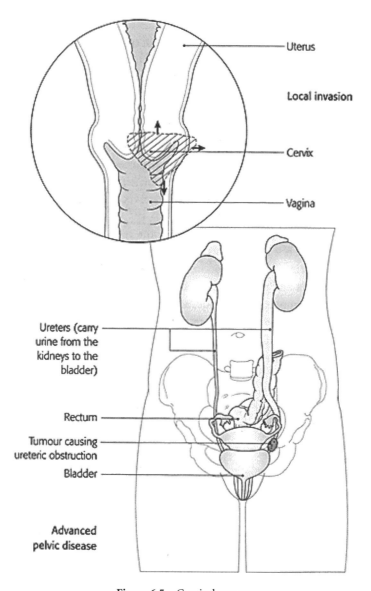

Figure 6.5   Cervical cancer

- There are two main types of cervical cancer. The first type grows in the skin lining the cervix. The second type grows from the lining of the mucous glands of the cervix. Most cervical cancers are associated with infection by a virus called HPV.
- Cervical cancer has two main ways of spreading: local invasion and lymphatic spread. The spread of cancer to different parts of the body is called metastasis.

Figure 6.5 (*Continue on facing page*)

- Local invasion means that the tumour grows into the upper vagina, the uterus and the tissue in the pelvis next to the uterus. In advanced cancer, the tumour may grow into the bladder at the front of the cervix and into the rectum at the back. It may also block the ureters, the tubes that carry urine from the kidneys to the bladder, causing kidney failure.
- Lymphatic spread occurs when cancerous cells move through the lymph fluid channels and are trapped by lymph glands, where the cells can multiply and form tumours.

pelvis. It usually involves you being taken to a theatre for an examination under anaesthetic (EUA), the procedure designed to stage your cancer. This is not in any way a curative procedure, but is designed to determine where the tumour is. This usually encompasses looking in the bladder (cystoscopy), looking in the vagina (colposcopy), looking in the rectum/colon (sigmoidoscopy), and taking appropriate biopsies. See Figure 6.6 for information on cystoscopy, biopsy and sigmoidoscopy.

Cervical cancer is also unique amongst the gynaecological cancers in that the staging is done before the potential curative surgery. All the other cancers are staged after the definitive surgery. This is because for many women the best treatment is not with surgery, but with chemo and radiotherapy. Staging is shown in Table 6.3.

All staging refers to the FIGO classification (Table 6.3). This stands for Federation Internationale Gynaecologie Oncologie; this is an international committee who have agreed upon the exact classification of each cancer in gynaecology. This is very important so that different hospitals, countries, etc. can compare their results for each cancer stage by stage. You can imagine that if somebody has a new idea for treating a type of cancer, it is terribly important to know which stages it is suitable for and to be able to assess if it works.

The FIGO staging is reproduced word for word and uses medical terminology. The medical terms are to be found in the glossary and also in the anatomy overview earlier in the book. **This staging is not in any way related to the 4 cusps (A–D).**

The treatment offered to you after the staging procedure will depend upon the stage that your cancer is at. If your cancer is stage IA1, then treatment is with a cone biopsy or simple hysterectomy, depending on whether

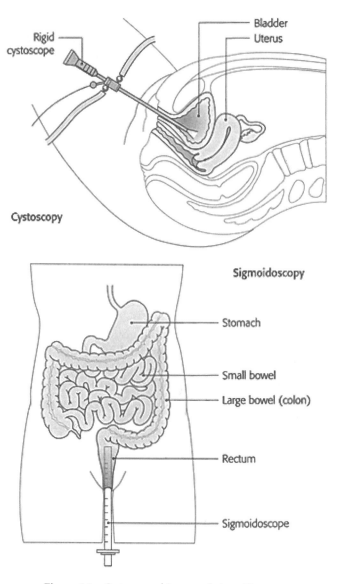

Figure 6.6   Cystoscopy, biopsy and sigmoidoscopy.

- Treatment of cervical cancer depends on the stage that the disease has reached (Table 6.3). This is a measure of the size of the tumour and how far it has spread. Your doctor may carry out several different investigations (including a thorough pelvic examination), often under general anaesthetic.
- A piece of tissue, called a biopsy, may be removed in the colposcopy clinic or while you are anaesthetised. This is then sent to the laboratory for analysis.

Figure 6.6 *(Continue on facing page)*

- Your bladder may be examined in a procedure called cystoscopy. A narrow telescope, called a cystoscope, is inserted into your urethra to examine the bladder for signs that it has been affected by the cancer. The urethra is the tube through which urine passes out of the body.
- The lower part of the bowel may be examined in a procedure called sigmoidoscopy. A metal or plastic tube, called a sigmoidoscope, is inserted into the back passage.
- After these investigations, you may feel some discomfort when you go to the toilet, but this should pass within a day or so.
- Many patients with cervical cancer do not need these investigations.

Table 6.3 FIGO staging of cervical cancer. (Stage 0 comes from TMN classification.)

Stage 0	Intra-epithelial neoplasia CIN 1, CIN 2, CIN 3
Stage I	The carcinoma is strictly confined to the cervix, extension to the uterine corpus should be disregarded.

Ia

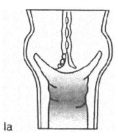

la

Preclinical carcinomas of the cervix (i.e., those diagnosed by microscopy only). All gross lesions, even with superficial invasion, are stage 1b. Invasion is limited to measured stromal invasion with a maximum depth of 5 mm and no wider than 7 mm. Measurement of the depth of invasion should be from the base of the epithelium, either surface or glandular, from which it originates. Vascular space involvement, either venous or lymphatic, should not alter the staging.

Ia1	Minimal microscopically evident stromal invasion. The stromal invasion is no more than 3 mm deep and no more than 7 mm in diameter.
Ia2	Lesions detected microscopically that can be measured. The measured invasion of the stroma is deeper than 3 mm but no greater than 5 mm, and the diameter is no wider than 7 mm.
Ib	Clinical lesions confined to the cervix, or preclinical lesions greater than stage 1a.
Ib1	

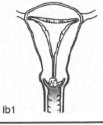

Clinical lesions less than 4 cm in size.

Ib1

(Continued)

Table 6.3   *(Continued)*

Ib2	Clinical lesions greater than 4 cm in size.
Stage II	Involvement of the vagina except the lower third, or infiltration of the parametrium. No involvement of the pelvic sidewall.

IIa

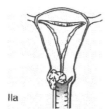

Involvement of the upper two-thirds of the vagina, but not out to the sidewall.

IIb

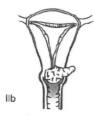

Involvement of the parametrium, but not out to the sidewall.

Stage III   Involvement of the lower third of the vagina. Extension to the pelvic sidewall. On rectal examination there is no cancer-free space between the tumour and the pelvic sidewall. All cases with a hydronephrosis or non-functioning kidney should be included, unless this is known to be attributable to another cause.

IIIa

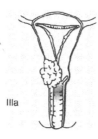

Involvement of the lower third of the vagina, but not out to the pelvic sidewall if the parametrium is involved.

IIIb

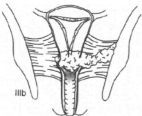

Extension onto the pelvic sidewall and/or hydronephrosis or non-functional kidney.

(Continued)

Table 6.3 (*Continued*)

Stage IV	Extension of the carcinoma beyond the reproductive tract.	

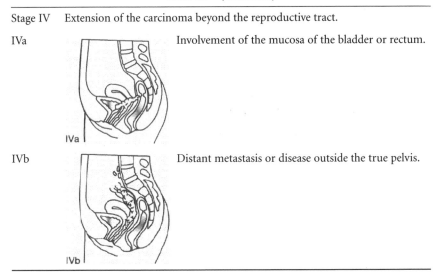

IVa — Involvement of the mucosa of the bladder or rectum.

IVb — Distant metastasis or disease outside the true pelvis.

you have finished your family or not, will be advised. The cure rate here is virtually 100%. Please see Figure 6.9 for a more in-depth description of a cone biopsy and simple hysterectomy.

Stage IA2 Cancer

The treatment of this type of cancer is highly specific to each patient. For some of you, treatment by cone biopsy alone may be the correct thing to do. For others, a radical hysterectomy (Figure 6.10) may be the correct thing to do and for others wishing to retain fertility, a procedure called radical trachelectomy (Figure 6.11) may be the appropriate operation. It may also be possible to do a cone biopsy and laparoscopic/robotic lymphadenectomy. If you are having fertility sparing surgery by way of trachelectomy (removal of the cervix and surrounding tissue, upper vagina and nodes), this may be done by a vaginal, abdominal, laparoscopic or robotic route. The choice will depend on your surgeon. These operations are described in Figures 6.10 and 6.11.

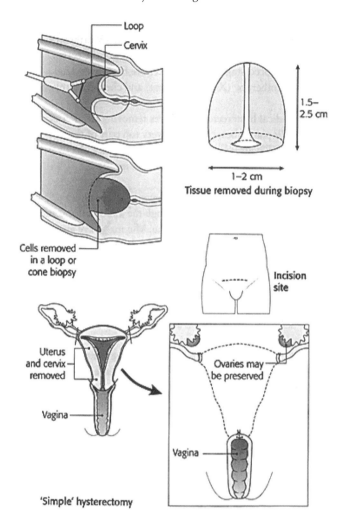

Figure 6.9   Loop biopsy, cone biopsy and simple hysterectomy.

- If a cervical cancer is at a very early stage, it may be possible to treat it by removing just the lower part of the cervix. This may be performed using an electrical current (or diathermy) in a procedure known as loop biopsy, or a laser or a knife, in a cone biopsy. It may be carried out using a local or a general anaesthetic.
- You are likely to notice some discharge and abnormal bleeding afterwards, and this may continue for several weeks. Although you can get back to normal the day after the operation, you need to give your cervix time to heal. Avoid using tampons, and do not

Figure 6.9 (*Continue on facing page*)

have penetrative sex for four weeks. If the bleeding is heavy or the discharge becomes offensive, see your doctor.

- Occasionally, women are advised to have a 'simple' hysterectomy, where the uterus and cervix are removed under general anaesthetic. However, this is a rare treatment for cervical cancer.
- Following simple hysterectomy, a catheter may be passed up the urethra into the bladder to drain off the urine, and another tube may drain any bleeding from your abdomen. These tubes may be left in place for 1–2 days.
- Afterwards, you will be given painkillers. Any non-dissolvable skin stitches or staples will be removed after 5–7 days. After six weeks your vagina will have healed fully and will function normally.

Stage IB1 Cancer

These cancers are usually managed by either radical hysterectomy or a radical trachelectomy, depending on whether you have completed your family. If you are having a radical trachelectomy, this may be done as a vaginal or abdominal procedure. If the cancer is greater than 2 cm in diameter, an abdominal approach should be utilised to maximise cure rate and preserve fertility. The abdominal route may be offered as an open, laparoscopic or robotic procedure dependent upon your surgeon. Radical hysterectomy does not necessarily entail removal of your ovaries and this is a separate issue, again depending upon your age.

Stage IB2 Cancer

These cancers are usually managed by radiotherapy and chemotherapy and, unfortunately, they are not normally regarded as safe options for preserving fertility. Radiotherapy and chemotherapy are described in detail in Chapter 12.

Stage IIA to IV Cancer

Stages IIA, IIB, IIIA, IIIB and IV are all also treated with chemotherapy and radiotherapy as described in Chapter 12.

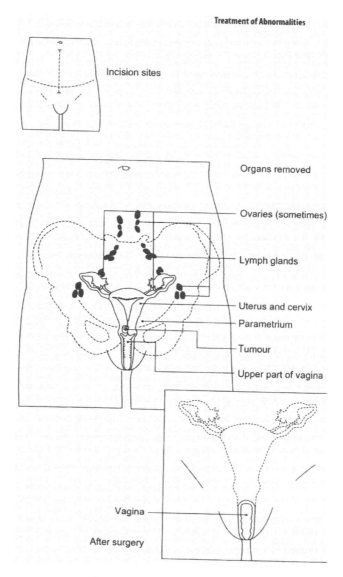

Figure 6.10   Radical hysterectomy.

- Radical hysterectomy, sometimes called Wertheim's hysterectomy, is performed for cancer of the cervix. Advanced stages of this cancer are best treated by radiotherapy (X-ray treatment) and chemotherapy.
- Radical hysterectomy involves removing the uterus, Fallopian tubes, cervix, the very top part of the vagina, lymph glands in the pelvis and, sometimes, the ovaries. The vagina may be shortened as a result.

Figure 6.10 *(Continue on facing page)*

- During the operation, a catheter is passed either up through the urethra or though the abdomen and into the bladder, to drain off the urine. You may have another tube in your abdomen or vagina to drain any slight bleeding. The catheter is usually left in for at least five days, and the other tube is usually left in place for 1–2 days. It sometimes takes several weeks before your bladder begins to work properly again, and changes in bladder sensation and function are sometimes permanent.
- You will be given painkillers to relieve the pain after the operation. Because your ovaries make the female hormones oestrogen and progesterone, you may also be prescribed hormone replacement therapy (HRT), if your ovaries have been removed.
- A course of radiotherapy and chemotherapy may be necessary after surgery.
- After the operation, avoid having penetrative sex for about six weeks to allow the top of the vagina to heal fully.

Surgical Procedures Referred to in this Chapter

	EUA: examination under anaesthetic (general)
Staging procedures:	Cystoscopy
	Sigmoidoscopy
	Colposcopy +/− Hysteroscopy
Treatment procedures:	Cryotherapy
	Lletz loop excision
	Cone biopsy
	Simple hysterectomy
	Radical hysterectomy: open, laproscopic, or robotic
	Radical trachelectomy — Vaginal
	Abdominal: open, laparoscopic or robotic

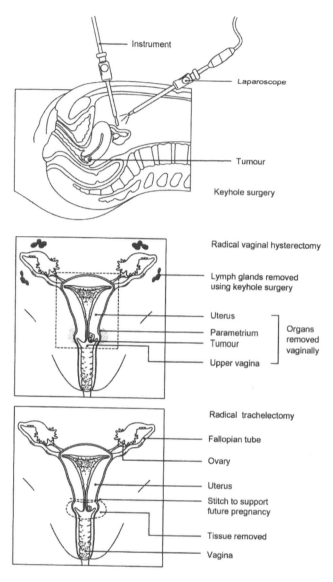

Instrument

Laparoscope

Tumour

Keyhole surgery

Radical vaginal hysterectomy

Lymph glands removed
using keyhole surgery

Uterus

Parametrium

Tumour

Upper vagina

Organs
removed
vaginally

Radical trachelectomy

Fallopian tube

Ovary

Uterus

Stitch to support
future pregnancy

Tissue removed

Vagina

Figure 6.11   Laparoscopically assisted radical vaginal hysterectomy and radical trachelectomy.

- Laparoscopically assisted radical vaginal hysterectomy and radical trachelectomy are newer alternatives to radical hysterectomy. Performed only in certain specialist centres, they are only suitable for small cancers. They are carried out under general anaesthetic.
- For these keyhole surgery procedures, a small cut is made in the belly button and the abdomen is filled with gas. A narrow telescope, called a laparoscope, is then inserted so

Figure 6.11   *(Continue on facing page)*

that the surgeon can see into the abdomen. Various keyhole surgery instruments are passed through other small cuts in the abdomen wall. The surgeon removes the lymph glands in the pelvis through the small cuts.

- In a laparoscopically assisted radical vaginal hysterectomy, the uterus, Fallopian tubes and, sometimes but not always, ovaries are initially freed from their attachments using the laparoscope. The uterus and its surrounding tissue, the cervix and the top part of the vagina are finally removed through the vagina.
- In radical vaginal trachelectomy, the cervix and upper part of the vagina are removed, but the uterus is left in place. The lymph glands in the pelvis are also removed, usually by keyhole surgery. This is only suitable for tumours caught in the early stage. As the uterus is left in place, you can, potentially, still become pregnant. A stitch is made at the bottom of the uterus, and this takes the place of the cervix in supporting a pregnancy. A baby would be delivered by Caesarean section.
- In radical abdominal trachelectomy, the cervix and lymph nodes are removed via an abdominal incision, thus allowing for a fertility sparing procedure for larger tumours.

Chapter 7

Ovarian Cancer including Cancer of the Fallopian Tube

This chapter covers the subject of ovarian cancer and Fallopian tube cancer. Fallopian tube cancer used to be thought of as a very rare condition and when it did arise, it appeared to follow a very similar course to that of ovarian cancer. However, since 2012 there have been new data that show that 70% of what were thought to be ovarian cancers, in fact have arisen within the Fallopian tube. They arise at the end of the tube closest to the ovary (distal end) and then it appears the early abnormal cells implant in the ovary, giving the impression that the cancer has arisen in the ovary. In practical terms this does not make for any difference in cancer management. They are 'staged' in the same way and are treated in the same way. The staging refers to how far the cancer has spread. Because of the great similarities, although the chapter refers to ovarian cancer, it also applies to Fallopian tube cancer. There will be no further mention made of Fallopian tube cancer in this chapter, but what is written here relating to ovarian cancer would apply to you if you have Fallopian tube cancer.

The only material difference lies in the area of prevention. We now know that whenever we remove ovaries to prevent ovarian cancer in the future, we must also strive to remove the Fallopian tubes at the same time. We have always routinely removed most of the tube anyway, and most importantly, we have always removed the 'important' end of the tube (i.e. the end closest to the ovary). We have, however, since 2012 striven to remove the whole tube and when we remove the uterus we remove the whole tube if we preserve the ovaries. We used to leave some of the tube attached to the ovaries but we now remove this as well to minimise the chances of ovarian/Fallopian cancer in the future.

General Facts

Of all the cancers affecting women, lymphoma and cancers of the breast, colon and uterus are more common than cancer of the ovary. Cancer of the ovary accounts for approximately one quarter of all gynaecological cancers. Overall the risk for women is approximately 1:70 of developing this type of tumour. It tends to occur most commonly between the ages of 55 and 59, but can occur at any age. It tends to be commoner in white women than black women. There has been an increasing incidence of this cancer over the last 40 years, which may come down to women having smaller families, increased affluence and an increasingly high fat diet. A number of things are associated with ovarian cancer and these include having never been pregnant, infertility, high fat diet, higher socio-economic status, family history, celibacy, early menopause, and exposure to talcum powder and asbestos. Ovarian cancer is also associated with breast and endometrial cancer and all three of these cancers are associated with high fat diet. There is possibly an association with ovarian stimulatory drugs, but there is certainly no evidence of an association between *in vitro* fertilisation (IVF) and ovarian cancer unless there have been multiple cycles. The only study showing this link suggested that there was an issue only in those who had more than 12 cycles of IVF. As might be expected, things which suppress egg production, namely the oral contraceptive pill and multiple pregnancies, are protective against ovarian cancer. **The oral contraceptive pill, if taken for five years continuously, gives a 40% reduction in the risk of ovarian cancer. If taken continuously for ten years, this rises to a 70% reduction. Starting and stopping the pill negates this benefit and is NOT advisable.**

Screening

Much effort is currently being made to develop a screening test for ovarian cancer. Screening programmes for cancer are ideal if they identify a change within an organ before cancer itself develops, and that this change is easily treated and for that matter, easily detected. For this reason, screening for cancer of the cervix is ideal because there is a pre-cancerous phase that takes up to two to three decades to develop into cancer and is easily detected by taking a smear. In addition, when the pre-cancer is found, it is safely and easily treated with a very high success rate.

In contrast, the mammogram programme for breast cancer is not designed to detect a pre-cancerous phase, but is designed to detect early cancer, the theory being that if you detect the cancer early, you are more likely to cure it than if you detect it late. It is therefore intrinsically not as good, some of the reason for all the negative press currently. It is still, however, the best test we have.

Both the breast and the cervix both have the advantage of being easily accessible. The breast can be investigated by examination and mammography, while the cervix can be smeared. One of the great difficulties with the ovary is that it is an internal organ and it is difficult to detect changes within it by examination alone. Also, to further complicate matters, the ovary is a naturally 'cystic' structure: it normally forms a cyst every month when it produces an egg, which is exactly what it is designed to do. If you scan women, most of them will have small ovarian cysts at one time or another and in fact every month in a woman who is fertile, follicles will be developing and will show as cysts on scans. After the eggs have been produced, a little cyst called the corpus luteum, which produces progesterone, the natural hormone to support pregnancy, will also be seen. This obviously means that if you utilise scanning to screen people for ovarian cysts, a very high number of the scans will show positive, whereas virtually none of these women will in fact have cancer.

A number of ways of screening for ovarian cancer have been investigated, including performing vaginal examination, performing ultrasound scans and measuring a blood test called CA-125. CA-125 is a protein that can be produced by ovarian cancer. It is, however, also produced in benign gynaecological conditions, such as endometriosis and fibroids, which further complicates matters. A new area of development is called proteomics, which is looking at detecting various proteins in the bloodstream that may be produced early on in the development of ovarian and other cancers. While this holds some promise, it is still far off from being used in clinical practice. Currently, if you are to be screened for ovarian cancer, this will encompass having ultrasound scans performed with the probe within the vagina (transvaginal ultrasound), coupled with measurements from blood tests of CA-125, coupled with vaginal examinations. Even combining these tests together carries a high false positive rate. This means that it is much more likely you will be told that you might have a cancer when in fact you don't and you would have to undergo surgical investigation to determine whether or not you have a cancer. At the moment, because of this high risk of subjecting women who have no problem to unnecessary surgery, screening is limited within the NHS in the UK to patients who have two close relatives (mother or sister) who have had ovarian cancer. In North America and the remainder of Western Europe and in private practice within the UK, having one close relative with ovarian cancer is usually seen as being adequate to commence screening, although gynaecologists may be placing their patients at increased risk and anxiety because of the high rate of over-diagnosis of the problem. For the most part, ovarian cancer, if it is detected, is detected in its true cancerous form, rather than in a pre-cancerous form. In other words, it is a bit like breast cancer where you aim to detect the cancer earlier rather than later and thus increase the cure rate.

There are two long running studies in the UK, the first for those women with a family history (UKFOCSS), and the other for those with no family history (UKCTOCS). The latter of these studies has yet been completed, but the 2014 guidelines based on UKFOCCSS are that for women with a family history (one or more close relatives), ultrasound and examination should take place once a year and CA-125 blood testing should take place twice a year. The absolute result of the CA-125 is not what matters; it is the trend over time. For example, the normal range is 1–36. If you have a measurement of 45, this does not mean you have cancer; this may be your norm. If, however, on repeat it had risen to 95, that would be more than double and therefore worrying. Conversely, if your first measurement is 5 (i.e., low), that is reassuring, but if the repeat was 12, still very much in the normal range, that would be worrying because it had more than doubled.

The results of the study for those with no family history (UKCTOCS) are eagerly awaited and due in 2015. For the time being, the standard practice is not to offer screening in the absence of a family history.

Until 2013, it was only possible to conduct genetic analyses if one could obtain blood from the 'index case' (i.e., your relative who had had cancer).

Very few people were therefore tested. However, it is now possible to test people in the absence of an index case. The tests are done for a number of gene mutations including BRCA1/2 and others. These mutations can give a high chance of breast, ovary or colon cancer. However, the 'golden rule' of all medical tests is to not do the test unless you know what you plan to do with the result, whatever it may be. Everybody hopes for a negative result and if this happens, all is well and good. If however the result is positive, one's strategy should be worked out before embarking on the tests. In addition, as well as the possibility of a positive and a negative test, there is a chance (10–15%) of you having a mutation of uncertain significance — i.e., you are not normal, but nobody knows what your mutation means. In addition, if you have a positive or equivocal test, this may then have ramifications for your children. Currently, insurance and mortgage companies do not ask about genetic testing when you apply for life insurance or a mortgage, but this is a voluntary moratorium. To do genetic testing with no index case in 2000 cost $380,000; the current price is $2,000 and falling. This means these tests will become much commoner and understanding will increase; however, our current advice is APPROACH WITH CAUTION!

What do I do with My Result?

If you have a positive result, in the case of breast cancer, this might involve having your breasts removed and/or your ovaries when you are in your forties. For women who have not had genetic testing, but have a strong family history of breast cancer, most will do an annual mammogram, breast examination and possibly breast ultrasound anyway. If this is all you would do after a positive genetic test, you could argue you would be better saving the £2000/$3000 doing the genetic tests and just do the screening anyway.

If you have a family history of ovary cancer, you may be doing the screening described above anyway (CA-125 twice yearly, ultrasound and examination once a year). You may also wish to have your ovaries and Fallopian tubes removed when you are past 40 years of age or to wait until the menopause to do this, depending upon what age your relatives them-selves were when they developed cancer. If you have a family history of breast cancer as well there is a greater drive to remove your ovaries in your early forties rather than wait until the menopause. Please note that the average age for the menopause is 51 years with a normal range of 40–56 years. Once you have your ovaries removed, you will go into menopause and even if there is a family history of breast cancer, you are best advised to take hormone replacement therapy (HRT) until the age of 50.

If you have been genetically tested for BRCA1 and are positive, prophylactic bilateral mastectomy is advised between the ages of 38–40. If you are BRCA2 positive, the procedure is advised between the ages of 40–45. The procedure is more effective for BRCA2 carriers, but overall this procedure may reduce your risk of breast cancer by up to 50%.

In addition, we know that in general actuarially women having a hysterectomy for benign causes who have their ovaries removed prophylactically to prevent ovarian cancer only get a life expectancy advantage if they take HRT. In addition to this, we know that women lose 50% of their bone mass within 20 years of the menopause and then are at risk of osteoporotic fracture. In a 70-year-old, a fractured neck of femur (hip) carries a 50% five-year death rate. This compares to a 30% five-year death rate in the woman newly diagnosed with breast cancer aged 70 years. Thus, before you decide what you want to do you should have a very comprehensive discussion with your doctor before embarking on your chosen route.

Types of Ovarian/Fallopian Tube Cancer

As well as cancer of these organs, there is a further disease which used to be seen as an intermediate form for problems in the ovary called 'borderline'. We used to believe that there was a 'sliding scale' where normal could go to borderline, which could then go on to become ovarian cancer. This is no longer thought to be the case. 'Borderline' is a separate entity and usually does not develop into cancer, although it brings its own problems. 'Borderline' is not a true cancerous state; in other words, it does not have the ability to spread, other than directly, but not through the bloodstream or through the lymph system.

Where patients have developed a cancer or borderline lesion, this is 'staged'. Staging refers to how far the tumour has spread and the following table with adjoining diagram shows a representation of this.

All staging refers to the FIGO classification (Table 7.1). This stands for Federation Internationale Gynaecologie Oncologie; this is an international

Table 7.1   FIGO staging of ovarian cancer.

Stage I	Tumour confined to ovaries	
Ia		Tumour limited to one ovary, capsule intact, no tumour on surface, negative washings.
Ib		Tumour involves both ovaries, otherwise like Ia.
Ic		Tumour limited to one or both ovaries. Surgical spill. Capsule rupture before surgery or tumour on ovarian surface. Malignant cells in the ascites or peritoneal washings.
Stage II	Tumour involves one or both ovaries with pelvic extension (below the pelvic brim) or primary peritoneal cancer.	
IIa		Extension and/or implant on uterus and/or Fallopian tubes.
IIb		Extension to other pelvic intraperitoneal tissues.
IIc		Tumour either stage IIa or b, but with ascites or positive peritoneal washings

(Continued)

Table 7.1   (*Continued*)

Stage III	Tumour involves one or both ovaries with cytologically or histologically confirmed spread to the peritoneum outside the pelvis and/or metastasis to the retroperitoneal lymph nodes.

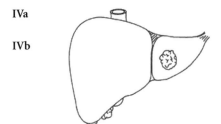

IIIa	Positive retroperitoneal lymph nodes and/or microscopic metastasis beyond the pelvis
IIIa1	Positive retroperitoneal lymph nodes only IIIa1(i) Metastasis ≤ 10 mm IIIa1(ii) > 10 mm
IIIa2	Microscopic, extrapelvic (above the brim) peritoneal involvement ± positive retroperitoneal lymph nodes.
IIIb	Microscopic, extrapelvic, peritoneal metastasis ≤ 2 cm ± positive retroperitoneal lymph nodes. Includes extension to capsule of liver/spleen.
IIIc	Microscopic, extrapelvic, peritoneal metastasis > 2 cm ± positive retroperitoneal lymph nodes. Includes extension to capsule of liver/spleen.
Stage IV	Distant metastasis excluding peritoneal metastasis
IVa	Pleural effusion with positive cytology.
IVb	Hepatic and/or splenic parenchymal metastasis, metastasis to extra-abdominal organs (including inguinal lymph nodes and lymph nodes outside of the abdominal cavity).

committee who have agreed upon the exact classification of each cancer in gynaecology. This is very important so that different hospitals, countries, etc. can compare their results for each stage. You can imagine that if somebody has a new idea for treating a type of cancer, it is terribly important to know which stages it is suitable for and to assess whether it works. The

FIGO staging is reproduced word for word and has very technical terms. These are explained in the glossary (pages 229 and 230) and in the anatomy overview (pages 7–10). This staging of ovarian cancer is determined by the results of the operation, which you may be about to undergo, or have undergone. **This staging (I–IV) is NOT in any way related to the cusps (A–D).**

Diagnosis

There are various routes by which you may have come to your gynaecological cancer specialist. This may be because you have felt a lump in your tummy, or on examination, a lump in your tummy has been found. It may also be that you have had a scan for one reason or another, which has detected a cyst on the ovary. When you arrive at the gynaecological cancer clinic, you will meet your gynaecological cancer specialist who will talk through with you the possibilities for treatment. He/she will wish to do blood tests. These will include tests for anaemia, tests of your blood salts, the function of your liver and your tumour markers. Tumour markers are blood tests that detect proteins produced by cancers and, in general, people will check for CA-125, which can go up with ovarian cancer, and also another marker called carcino embryonic antigen (CEA). This tends to be raised with bowel cancer. They may also test for CA 19-9, a marker which may rise with ovary, colon, pancreatic and appendix tumours. This marker rises in the presence of mucous-secreting tumours.

The specialist will perform an examination of your tummy and pelvis and perhaps take a cervical smear, if you have not had this done recently. They will then order a CT scan of your chest and abdomen and possibly an MRI scan to further determine how things are in your pelvis and abdomen. If you have not had an ultrasound scan, they will arrange this too.

In general, we utilise a formula called the risk of malignancy index (RMI) (Table 7.2). This is a way of determining whether women have a high chance that any cyst on their ovary is benign or whether it might be cancerous. If the risk of malignancy index is less than 200, this is regarded as a good result and if it is more than 200, then one has to tread more cautiously.

The risk of malignancy index encompasses a score that is related to your menopause. If you are before the menopause, then you score one, and if you are after the menopause, you score three. It also relates to the findings

Table 7.2 Table of RMI, <200 is reassuring, >200 requires further investigation.

CA-125	×	ultrasound findings	×	menopause status
(1–36 = normal range)		(0 = no cyst, 1 = cyst with one feature, or 3 = cyst with more than one feature)		(1 = not menopausal, or 3 = menopausal)

on your ultrasound scan, for which again you may score one or three. Finally, it also relates to your CA-125 level. To find your risk of malignancy index (RMI), we multiply your CA-125 level times your ultrasound findings score times your menopause status score. As you can imagine, if you are before the menopause and have a simple-looking cyst, then you must have a very high CA-125 for there to be a problem. If you are after the menopause and have a complicated cyst, you would only need to have a relatively low CA-125 to jump the threshold for the cyst requiring to be managed as if it were a cancer, even although it may well not be.

If you are somebody who has a risk of malignancy index of less than 200, then if you are before the menopause, you may well be eligible for management by keyhole surgery. If, however, the risk of malignancy index is over 200, it is still very possible that you do not have a cancer, but nobody can take a chance on this. If you have an ovary with cancer cells in it and, as you can imagine, under keyhole management where the cyst has burst, these cancerous cells could then spread around the inside of your abdomen/tummy and spread the cancer. This would make a stage Ia cancer, which is quite curable by surgery alone, into a stage Ic cancer, which is still quite curable, but requires to have chemotherapy as well as surgery.

Unfortunately, therefore, if your risk of malignancy index is over 200, you have to be managed as if you may have a cancer. This means that you are required to be properly 'staged' and the ovary which has the problem in it requires to be removed intact. This usually requires a midline opening of your tummy (midline laparotomy), as shown in Figure 7.1. Sometimes, with the development of new bags for retrieving ovaries, it may be possible to remove the ovary laparoscopically (i.e. keyhole), analyse it intra-operatively, a technique called 'frozen section', and then decide whether to do an open procedure. One can also sample the omentum and lymph nodes laparoscopically if required. The newer bags are much more robust than the older ones and, therefore, reliably do not burst or leak. Having said all of this, the majority of patients will require an open procedure.

If you are somebody who has a scan which suggests that there may be cancer that has spread outside the ovary, then you will also be required to have a midline opening of your tummy (midline laparotomy). This is designed to determine how much cancer is inside your abdomen and to remove as much of it as is possible.

There are four potential outcomes under this circumstance. One is that the tumour is completely removed so that there is no visible tumour left to the naked eye (complete macroscopic clearance of the tumour, no residual disease (R zero)). This is the best result and one your surgeon will strive for. The second potential outcome is that the cancer is removed to the extent that there is no cancer left in your abdomen that is greater than 1 cm diameter in size (see Figure 7.1); this is called an optimal debulk. The third potential outcome is that a lot of cancer is removed, but there are still areas of tumour greater than 1–2 cm in size. This, with modern scanning and surgical techniques, is unlikely. The fourth potential outcome is that the tumour is completely irremovable. The last eventuality that the tumour is not removable at all is extremely unlikely. Clearly, the first option is the best and the fourth option is the worst. The reason for this, apart from being self-evident, relates to how well chemotherapy will work for you. If there is only microscopic disease left, the chemotherapy has a better chance of clearing it than if there are small lumps of cancer left. In turn, the chemotherapy is better at dealing with small lumps of tumour than large ones. In recent years, we now know that greater surgical effort pays off. If you can leave no residual disease in the abdomen and pelvis, the patient will do much better. If before your surgeon operates, he/she suspects that the latter two options are possible, they will not operate but refer you to the medical oncologists for chemotherapy first. You will get three pulses of chemotherapy and then be rescanned and then assessed again as to whether your tumour is removable surgically. If it is, all is well and good; if it is not, you will be given a further three pulses of chemotherapy and the scans then again repeated. If the tumour has now become removable, you will be offered surgery. After the surgery, you will get a further three pulses of chemotherapy. If it is not removable, you will be offered further chemotherapy.

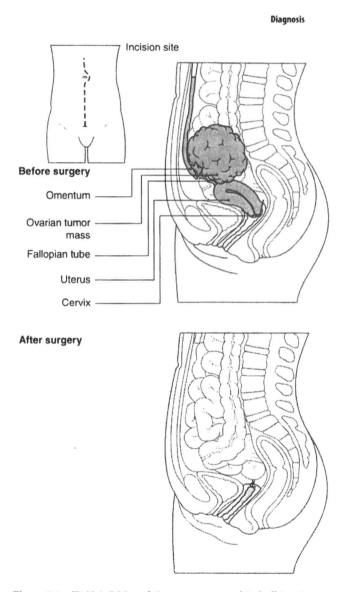

Figure 7.1   TAH & BSO and Omentectomy, and Debulking Surgery.

- If your ovarian cancer is at an early stage, you will probably have a total abdominal hysterectomy and bilateral salpingo-oophorectomy (TAH & BSO). This involves removing the uterus, cervix, Fallopian tubes and ovaries. The pelvic lymph glands may also be removed. The fat 'apron' in the abdomen (the omentum) is also removed in a procedure called omentectomy.

Figure 7.1 *(Continue on facing page)*

- The operation is carried out under general anaesthetic. A catheter will drain urine from the bladder for a few days, and you will stay in hospital for up to one week.

- Your doctor may not know whether your tumour is benign or cancerous or, if cancerous, how advanced it is, until the pathology report is available, usually 7–14 days after the operation.

- If the cancer is advanced, it is necessary to remove as much of the tumour as possible during the operation; this is called debulking surgery, and may involve bowel surgery. This does not cure ovarian cancer, but can delay or prevent complications, such as bowel or kidney obstruction. It also makes chemotherapy, which is treatment with drugs that attack the cancer cells, more effective.

- If the cancer affects only one ovary, and you have yet to complete your family, a unilateral oophorectomy may be an option. This involves removing only the affected ovary. You may be recommended to have the other ovary removed with a hysterectomy later.

Surgery for Ovarian Cancer

Post Menopause/Family Completed

You will have midline laparotomy (i.e., your tummy will be opened through a vertical incision) (see Figure 7.1). You will have a hysterectomy, either total or subtotal, which is explained on pages 70 and 71. You will have removal of the Fallopian tubes and both ovaries. In addition, the omentum, which is a fatty tissue that hangs from your stomach and transverse colon, will be removed. I have never met any patient who has ever heard of the omentum unless they were either a doctor, nurse or vet (see Figure 7.1). It is known as the 'abdominal policeman' because it goes to where trouble is. Unfortunately, therefore, in the case of cancers, it goes to the cancer and picks up cancer cells, which is why it is an early place for the spread of cancer. It therefore requires removal. Prior to the surgical era (before 1900), the omentum could prove to be important if, for instance, one developed appendicitis. It is difficult to imagine that appendicitis, which is now such an easily treated condition, before 1900 and before surgery carried such a high chance of dying. The omentum did protect people at that time, although even with your omentum, there was still an approximately 25% chance of dying. Nowadays, your omentum is something that you can certainly afford to lose. In addition, having removed the uterus, tubes and omentum, many surgeons will have an analysis made of the tissues which are removed while you are still in the theatre (frozen section). If there is a possibility that your cancer is confined to only one or two ovaries, they will then sample your lymph nodes along the main blood vessel, in the abdomen, the aorta and from alongside the vessels in the pelvis. Your surgeon may also remove your appendix. All of this is designed to be absolutely certain as to how far the cancer has spread. The rationale behind this is that if you have a cancer that is confined to one ovary and it truly is confined to that ovary, then the only treatment that you may need is surgery, which will confer a very high cure rate. If, however, the cancer has spread and if you don't take the right samples, you can't know whether the cancer has spread or not, and then you would also be required to be treated with chemotherapy.

For those women who have disseminated cancer — in other words, it has spread outside the ovary — every effort will be made to remove (debulk) it. This may require to have some bowel removed and for this reason you will have had your bowel prepared before the operation with a drink/enema to empty it. This is designed to minimise the risk of colostomy where the bowel is diverted into a bag. This is a relatively rare occurrence.

There is a new device called a PlasmaJet®, which allows the tumour to be removed from the bowel without damage to it. This increases the chance of tumour resection and minimises the chance of bowel resection.

Pre-Menopause/Family not Completed

If you have not completed your family, fertility sparing surgery may be possible. This depends on what the pre-operative investigations suggest. In addition, analyses can be undertaken during the operation (frozen section) to determine whether the tumour is benign, borderline or cancerous, and if borderline or cancerous, how far it has spread. Frozen section is fairly reliable, but not 100%. In other words, occasionally, the frozen section says there is no cancer and later it is discovered there is. It is rarely the other way around; if the frozen section is positive for cancer, it almost always is.

If your RMI lies below 200, all is well and good; it is highly unlikely that you have a cancer and fertility sparing surgery is the order of the day possibly via a keyhole approach. If, however it is above this, then you will require to be managed as if you have a cancer, even though you may not have. Remember the best result at the end is that it is benign; this does not mean that you have had unnecessary surgery.

If the scans done pre-operatively suggest that the tumour is confined to the ovary, you will be offered a midline laparotomy, removal of the affected ovary and adjoining Fallopian tube. This will then be analysed during your operation (frozen section). While the pathologist is doing the analysis, the omentum is removed. If there are any other suspicious areas, these will be biopsied. There are three possible results from the frozen section: benign, borderline or cancer. If benign or borderline, the procedure will stop at this point. If it is cancer, then your surgeon will proceed to sample your para-aortic and pelvic lymph nodes and possibly biopsy the other ovary. Your appendix may also be removed. The procedure will then finish and you will have retained your fertility organs. There is a very small chance that the full histology results, which will be available one week later, may necessitate further surgery, but this is very unlikely, and a chance many women believe is worth taking.

If the pre-operative scans suggest tumours in both ovaries, they would both require frozen section and may both have to be removed. This still leaves the possibility of retaining the uterus, which would allow pregnancy with donated eggs at a future date. Unfortunately, if ovarian cancer is diagnosed, it is not possible to store eggs/ovarian tissue, since IVF at a future date may result in re-implanting the cancer as well as the eggs. Finally, if the scans suggest disseminated cancer, then assuming frozen section analysis is positive for cancer, it will prove necessary to remove all the organs as in the operation described above for the post-menopausal woman. Thankfully, this is very uncommon but removes all chance of child bearing.

Post-Operative Care

Your surgeon will come and tell you what they've found within the first 24–48 hours after the operation. They will have much more data for you approximately 2–3 weeks later, when the results of all the samples removed have gone to the laboratory and been analysed. It is only at this stage then that the true stage, as shown on pages 83 and 84, of your cancer will be known.

If you have a stage Ia cancer, which does not appear aggressive in terms of its type, then no further active treatment will be given to you and you will be followed up with regular hospital visits for the next 5–10 years.

This follow up usually involves 3–4 monthly visits to the clinic with measurements of blood tests and examination of your abdomen/tummy and pelvis/vaginal examination coupled with blood tests and perhaps intermittent scans. It is terribly important to remember that 'one off' blood test results don't mean anything. It is trends that matter. Where there are blips up and down of CA-125, this does not matter. However, where CA-125 keeps rising, this is significant. Unfortunately for the person in the latter category, this means that they perhaps have a recurrence of their cancer, whereas blips Stage Ia higher grade up and down are not usually significant.

For the person with stage Ib or greater, where the cancer has spread out of the ovary, then further management is always suggested and has been shown to be beneficial. These days, some patients with stage Ia disease will also be offered chemotherapy.

Further management is usually with chemotherapy, but occasionally can be with radiotherapy. I would suggest that you go to Chapter 12 for more information on chemotherapy and radiotherapy if this applies to you. For the person who requires further management, the follow up is again similar, with review every 3–4 months for the first two years, then every six months for the next three years and then every year for the following five years. **I would also suggest that if you have had or are going to have chemotherapy, you refer to Chapter 1 on the 4 cusp approach, since much of this chapter relates to people in this position.**

Chapter 8

Endometrial Cancer

General Facts

Cancer of the endometrium is the most common gynaecological cancer and, in fact, the fourth most common cancer in women. It is $1\frac{1}{2}$ times as common as ovarian cancer and three times as common as cervical cancer. It would appear that since the 1970s, the number of women with endometrial cancer has risen, but commensurate with this rise has been a rise in the cure rate. This may be because of increasing awareness amongst women that when they have bleeding, particularly after their menstrual periods are finished, it is important that they attend their doctor for investigations. This has allowed earlier diagnosis of the condition and, as with all cancers, the usual rule is that the earlier you diagnose it, the higher the cure rate. Most women tend to be diagnosed between the age of 50 and 60, but 20–25% will have a diagnosis made before the menopause and a small percentage (5%) will be diagnosed before the age of 40. This is why for those women who have menstrual upset, particularly when they are in their forties, investigation is always undertaken to make sure that they don't have endometrial cancer. The vast majority of people with menstrual upset do not have endometrial cancer, but unfortunately a small minority do. Even when women who are in the menopause start bleeding again, the majority of these women do not have endometrial cancer, although clearly investigation has to be done to make certain that this is not the diagnosis.

In terms of lifestyle issues that have effects on the development of endometrial cancer, the oral contraceptive pill and cigarette smoking appear to reduce the risk, though this is not a reason to start smoking! While being overweight, never having been pregnant and a late menopause all tend to increase the risk.

In addition, the use of oestrogen-only hormone replacement therapy (HRT) without any progesterone causes an increased risk. If you have a uterus, most HRTs are prescribed with progesterone as well as oestrogen, unless you have had a hysterectomy. The progesterone may be given by tablets or maybe via a Mirena coil. Ironically, the risk of breast cancer is lower with oestrogen-only preparations than with combined ones. Unfortunately, it does not appear that the Mirena reduces the risk of breast cancer compared to oral progesterones. This is not what one would have expected. For women who have a uterus, some progesterone is usually used, although a few women choose to take oestrogen-only preparations, in the knowledge that they are increasing their risk of endometrial cancer while relatively reducing their risk of breast cancer. To put this into figures, a 50-year-old woman has a risk of breast cancer of 4.5%. If she takes oestrogen-only HRT for ten years, this will rise by 0.7% to 5.2%. If she takes combined HRT, the rise will be 1.8%; thus, her risk after ten years of usage will be 6.3%. However, the woman who has taken HRT has a higher cure rate for her breast cancer than the one who hasn't. This stems from two factors: women on HRT have their breasts more closely monitored, and they also tend to develop oestrogen-sensitive tumours, which intrinsically carry a higher cure rate.

There is an association of endometrial cancer with diabetes mellitus. Tamoxifen therapy, which is given to women with breast cancer, also unfortunately increases the risk of endometrial cancer. It is terribly important to say that in terms of risks versus benefits, if one has had breast cancer and is prescribed Tamoxifen therapy, the very small risk of getting endometrial cancer is very much outweighed by the reduced risk of getting one's breast cancer back, and **therefore, it is vitally important to take the Tamoxifen therapy that has been prescribed.**

Endometrial cancer happily carries a very high cure rate and while nobody would ever want to develop any form of cancer, there is no doubting that an endometrial cancer that is detected early has close to 100% cure

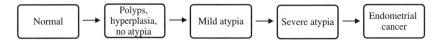

Figure 8.1   Sliding scale from normal to endometrial cancer.

rate. Mercifully, many women are diagnosed early and hence the prognosis is excellent, with relatively simple therapy for the majority.

Many women believe that when they go for investigation for bleeding, there are in essence two possibilities with respect to their diagnosis: one is that they have a benign condition and the other is that they have a cancerous condition. This is not the case with endometrial problems. There is effectively a sliding scale of abnormality, which starts with normal and moves to hyperplasia — in other words, cellular thickening of the endometrium. This thickening can have cells which are abnormal (the medical term being atypia) and which are graded mild, moderate or severe. Finally, at the end of this sliding scale is endometrial cancer. This is shown in Figure 8.1. In terms of treatment, simple thickening (hyperplasia) and hyperplasia with mild to moderate atypia (Figure 8.2) can all be treated medically with progesterone therapy. Progesterone is a hormone that occurs naturally in women in the second half of their cycle, after they have produced an egg, and this drug can be used to stabilise the lining of the uterus, namely the endometrium. It can either be administered in tablet form or via the Mirena coil. For the more severe forms of atypia, surgical management in the form of hysterectomy is usually advocated since, for a woman with severe atypia, she has a 50% chance of developing an endometrial cancer in two years if she is left untreated. For a woman wishing to preserve fertility, other options may be possible, but are not without some element of risk and these are discussed later.

How is the Diagnosis Made?

For a woman who is past menopause, the development of bleeding will alert her to the fact that she should go to her doctor. Her doctor will refer her rapidly to a gynaecologist for investigation of this bleeding. For women who are prior to the menopause, the usual method of being alerted is

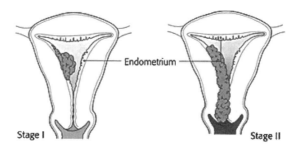

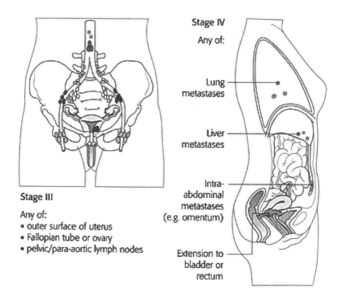

Figure 8.2   Endometrial cancer.

- The endometrium is the tissue that lines the uterus. Endometrial cancer usually occurs in women after the menopause, causing vaginal bleeding, though it can occur before the menopause, causing bleeding between periods.
- Endometrial cancer is often triggered by a hormone imbalance. Hormones are the chemical messengers that regulate the body's functions. Women have two main reproductive hormones, called oestrogen and progesterone. Progesterone, the hormone released when a woman ovulates, helps to protect against endometrial cancer. Progesterone is also present in hormonal contraceptives including the pill.
- A pre-cancerous form exists, called atypical endometrial hyperplasia. Depending on how abnormal the cells are, this can be treated with progesterone therapy or hysterectomy.

irregularity of her periods. Clearly, the majority of women coming up to the menopause tend to get some irregularity, which means that the vast majority of people who do get irregularity do not have cancer. It has to be said that the bleeding tends to be heavier and more frequent rather than less frequent in women who may have endometrial cancer. Most women going towards the menopause tend to have less frequent bleeding, rather than more frequent bleeding. A number of women are diagnosed as having endometrial cancer from their cervical smear. Although the cervical smear programme is not in any way designed to detect endometrial cancer, it does sometimes pick up abnormal cells from the endometrium.

In the past, when one arrived at the gynaecologist, the investigation that was performed was a D&C, which stands for dilatation and curettage (Figure 8.3). Dilatation refers to dilatation (opening) of the cervix and curettage refers to the process of scraping the inside of the uterus. This has not been regarded for many years as a proper investigation for endometrial cancer unless it is combined with the investigation of hysteroscopy (Figure 8.3). Hysteroscopy is where a small (3 mm wide) telescope is passed up through the cervix and into the inside of the uterus, allowing visualisation of the inside of the uterus. Hysteroscopy may be performed in the outpatient department under local anaesthetic, or in the operating theatre, usually as a day case procedure performed under general anaesthetic. Practice as to whether it is done as an inpatient or outpatient varies from hospital to hospital. Certainly, if it proved impossible to insert the telescope in the outpatient department, then admission will be arranged on another day to the operating theatre for the hysteroscopy under general anaesthetic. When that is done, the cervix requires dilatation and once one has seen what is inside the uterus, curettage is performed to obtain a sample to send to the laboratory (see Figure 8.3).

The alternative to hysteroscopy and D&C is outpatient sampling using a pipelle sampler (see Figure 8.4). This allows cells to be sucked up from inside the uterus and sent to the laboratory for analysis. This is a syringe-like device in the form of a thin tube with a suction mechanism. There is no needle. It is a 'blind' procedure, where the doctor cannot see where the sample is being taken from, and for this reason, an ultrasound scan is also performed. The ultrasound scan allows the doctor to assess the size of your uterus, the size of your ovaries and the thickness of your endometrium.

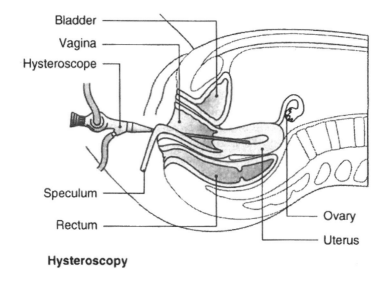

Hysteroscopy

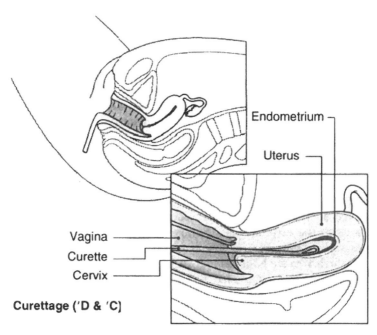

Curettage ('D & 'C)

Figure 8.3   Hysteroscopy and curettage.

- Hysteroscopy is a method of examining the uterus using a small telescope called a hysteroscope. It may be carried out under local anaesthetic in the outpatient clinic, or as a day-case procedure under general anaesthetic. It takes about 20 minutes.

Figure 8.3 *(Continue on facing page)*

- If you are awake, you will be asked to lie on your back with your legs in supports. The hysteroscope is passed though the vagina and cervix into the uterus. Gas or liquid is used to distend the uterus slightly to make the examination easier.
- A tissue sample or biopsy can be taken through some hysteroscopes. Alternatively, an endometrial biopsy device can be used, or the lining of the uterus can be scraped using an instrument called a curette (this is commonly known as a D&C). The tissue sample is sent for analysis.
- You may feel some discomfort similar to period pain for a few hours after hysteroscopy. You may also have a small amount of bleeding that lasts for 1–2 days.

If the endometrium is thin (less than 4 mm), it is highly unlikely that an endometrial cancer is present. If the endometrial thickness is great (more than 12 mm), either post-period or post-menopause, this is suspicious, and if there is nothing obtained on the outpatient sample, then you would be referred for a hysteroscopy to confirm that everything was okay. The trouble with outpatient sampling is that if no sample is obtained, and the bleeding continues or something is found on the sample, then the next investigation is to go for hysteroscopy and D&C. For this reason, many gynaecologists will decide and advise you to go straight for the hysteroscopy and D&C, rather than doing outpatient sampling coupled with ultrasound. As can be seen from all that I have written above, there is quite a lot of variation as to how different doctors investigate. It suffices to say though, that all are designed to maximise your safety.

As shown in Figure 8.2 the scope of what may be detected is quite wide. Polyps are fleshy growths which can arise in the endometrium or in the cervix. (They can also arise in your nose, in your throat, in your guts, etc.) The majority of polyps are benign, but having said this some may have atypical changes as in Figure 8.2 and very rarely may they prove to be cancerous.

What happens once the Diagnosis of Cancer is Made?

Having had the diagnosis of cancer made by your gynaecologist, a number of investigations will then follow. You will have blood taken to check that you are not anaemic, to check your blood salts (urea and electrolytes) and to check your liver function tests. You will almost certainly have an

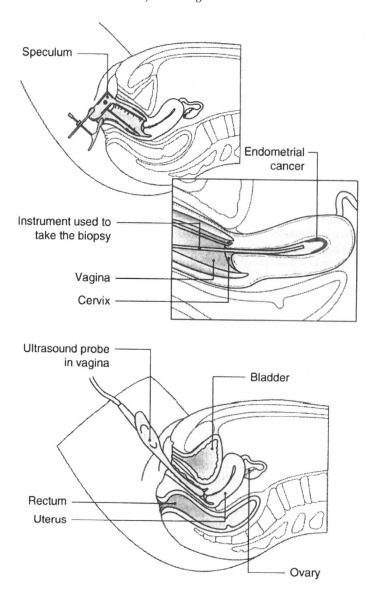

Figure 8.4   Endometrial biopsy and ultrasound.

- Endometrial biopsy and ultrasound can both be used to investigate the cause of abnormal bleeding.
- An endometrial biopsy is a sample of tissue taken from the lining of the uterus, known as the endometrium. The biopsy is usually carried out as an outpatient procedure without an anaesthetic.

Figure 8.4 (*Continue on facing page*)

- You will be asked to lie on your back with your legs apart. A plastic or metal instrument called a speculum is inserted into the vagina to hold the vaginal walls apart. A narrow plastic device is then passed into the vagina, through the cervix and into the uterus, where it is used to remove a piece of tissue. This is then sent to the laboratory.
- Endometrial biopsy is not usually painful. If you have not been pregnant, however, your cervix might be tightly closed. If this is the case, local anaesthetic can be used to numb the cervix, and a metal instrument can be used to open it gently. Sometimes, a general anaesthetic is needed.
- You can get back to normal straight away after an endometrial biopsy, but you may have spotting of blood for a few days afterwards. Laboratory results should be with your doctor in about a week.
- With ultrasound, a probe is gently placed in the vagina, and the image of the uterus is seen on a screen. Scan results are available immediately, but you may have to wait for your doctor to interpret them and inform you.

electrocardiogram (ECG) to check your heart and you will have blood taken for cross-match so that if you bleed during surgery, blood is available for you. In addition, another kind of X-ray investigation, probably a CT of your chest and abdomen and an MRI scan of your pelvis will take place.

All cancers are staged and the staging is called FIGO staging. FIGO (Federation Internationale Gynaecologique Oncologie) is an international committee who have agreed upon the exact classification of gynaecological cancers. It is very important so that different hospitals, countries, etc. can compare their results for each cancer, stage for stage. You can imagine that if somebody has a new idea for treating a type of cancer, it is terribly important to know which stage it is suitable for and to assess whether it works. Table 8.1 and Figure 8.2 shows the FIGO staging of endometrial cancer. If you look at older websites and books, it is important that you know this classification changed in 2009. **The FIGO staging I–IV has NO relationship to the 4 cusps A–D.**

Although the exact stage of your cancer can only be known after your surgery, we try very hard with our pre-operative investigations to get a good idea as to what stage your cancer is at before we take you to the operating theatre. This allows us to tailor your treatment to the presumed stage you are at. However, the actual stage of your cancer is only known after you have

Table 8.1   FIGO staging of endometrial cancer. (Stage 0 is from TMN staging.)

Stage	Criteria
	Primary tumour cannot be assessed
	No evidence of primary tumour
0	Carcinoma *in situ*
I	Tumour confined to uterine body
IA	Tumour limited to endometrium or involves <50% of myometrium
IB	Tumour invades ≥50% of endometrium
II	Tumour invades cervical stroma, does not extend beyond uterus
III	Local and/or regional spread of tumour
IIIA	Tumour invades serosa of uterine body/or adnexae
IIIB	Vaginal and/or parametrial involvement
IIIC	Metastases to pelvic and/or para-aortic lymph nodes
	IIIC1 positive pelvic nodes
	IIIC2 positive para-aortic lymph nodes with/without positive pelvic lymph nodes
IV	Tumour invdades bladder mucosa and/or bowel mucosa and/or distant metastases
IVA	Tumour invasion of bladder and/or bowel mucosa
IVB	Distant metastases, including intra-umbilical metastases and/or inguinal lymph nodes

had surgery. The mainstay of surgical treatment is an operation called a total hysterectomy and bilateral salpingo-oophorectomy. This means removal of your uterus, cervix, Fallopian tubes and ovaries. This operation is shown pictorially in Figure 8.5. Most surgeons perform this procedure laparoscopically, either as a total laparoscopic hysterectomy and bilateral salpingo oophorectomy (TLH, BSO) or a laparoscopically assisted vaginal hysterectomy and bilateral salpingo oophorectomy (LAVH, BSO). This is shown in Figure 8.5. Occasionally an open procedure may be required, but if you are heavily overweight the evidence strongly points to utilising a keyhole method. Sometimes these procedures are performed with robotic assistance.

There are debates amongst gynaecologists as to whether other things should be removed at the same time as the uterus, tubes and ovaries. This partly depends upon the estimate as to the stage of your cancer from the scans and blood tests which have been performed, and also may partly depend upon the centre at which you are being managed. There is agreement that for the earliest cancers, stage Ia, with no adverse features, a simple hysterectomy and removal of tubes and ovaries alone is adequate treatment. For cancers that have spread into the muscle of the uterus or elsewhere, there is debate as to whether it is valuable to remove the lymph glands at the same time as removing the uterus. Removal of the lymph glands is shown in Figure 8.5. In addition, some surgeons believe that it is better to just sample the lymph nodes so that if they are found to be positive, then you would be referred for further treatment. Other surgeons go for a more aggressive approach and remove all of the lymph nodes in the hope that this may improve the cure rate.

We, the authors, practice the latter approach if the patient is generally fit enough. As you can imagine, the fact that there are several different approaches means that nobody in truth actually knows the right answer as to what should be done, and for this reason there are a number of studies currently running within the UK, Europe and in the USA to try and answer these questions.

In addition to the lymph nodes, depending on the tumour type, surgeons will advocate removal of the omentum, which most people haven't heard of, but is a fatty structure that hangs from the stomach and transverse colon and is also called the 'abdominal policeman'. It gets this nickname because it goes to where the trouble is. Unfortunately, if one has a cancer, the omentum has a tendency to pick up cancer cells, and if cancer develops in the omentum, this means that there is spread outside the uterus and, therefore, the hysterectomy alone will not have worked as treatment.

For those women who have negative nodes — in other words, no spread to the lymph glands, and where the muscle of the uterus (myometrium) is only invaded to less than 50%, (stage Ia) — usually no further therapy is planned. For more advanced stages, follow up treatment with radiotherapy (external beam and vault brachytherapy) and possibly chemotherapy is standard if the lymph nodes have not been removed. If the lymph nodes have all been removed (i.e., not sampled), then chemotherapy with localised radiotherapy to the top of the vagina (vault brachytherapy) may be used.

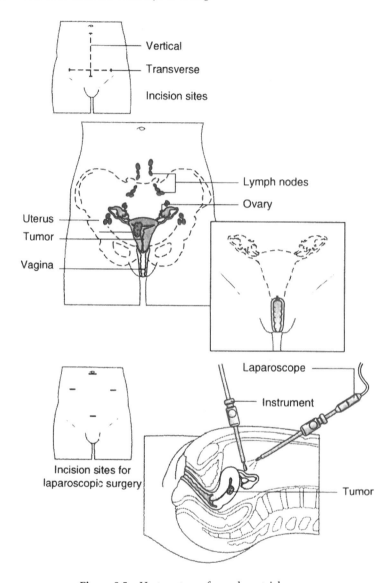

Figure 8.5　Hysterectomy for endometrial cancer.

- The usual operation for endometrial cancer involves removing the uterus, cervix, both Fallopian tubes and ovaries. The procedure is called a total abdominal hysterectomy and bilateral salpingo-oophorectomy (TAH & BSO for short).
- Sometimes, it is also necessary to remove the fat 'apron' in the abdomen (called the omentum), in a procedure called omentectomy. Similarly, the lymph glands in the pelvis may be removed.

Figure 8.5 *(Continue on facing page)*

- The operation is carried out under general anaesthetic, sometimes through a vertical (midline) or transverse (bikini-line) incision. A catheter may be passed up the urethra into the bladder to drain off the urine, and another tube may be inserted into the abdomen or vagina to drain any bleeding in the pelvis. These tubes may be left in place for 1–2 days.
- More commonly, the hysterectomy is performed using keyhole surgery. A narrow telescope called a laparoscope is inserted through a small cut in the belly button. Keyhole surgery instruments are inserted into the abdomen through other small cuts in the abdominal wall. The laparoscope is used to perform the early steps of the hysterectomy, and the organs are finally removed through the vagina. Lymph glands in the pelvis can also be removed using the laparoscope.

Radiotherapy

When radiotherapy is given, it may be given intra-vaginally (vault brachytherapy) or it may be given through the abdomen (external beam radiotherapy). If you might be going for radiotherapy or wish to find out more about this, go to Chapter 12.

Fertility Sparing Treatments for Endometrial Cancer

Until a few years ago, all of the treatments for endometrial cancer unfortunately involved loss of the ability to have children, because the treatment always encompassed removing the uterus. However, in the last few years, if a woman who has no children presents to her gynaecologist with an early stage endometrial cancer, discussion may take place about other options. Any woman whose cancer is invading into the muscle of the uterus unfortunately still has no other option but to go forward for hysterectomy. However, for women who have a stage Ia cancer, in other words, where the cancer is in the lining of the uterus, in the endometrium alone, it is possible to curette, in other words, scrape the tumour off, and then commence progesterone therapy in tablet form. There were descriptions in the past of use of the Mirena intrauterine device; however, this is now known not to be as effective as oral progesterone therapy. It is very important to say that if your gynaecologist starts this discussion with you, they will explain to you that the standard treatment has to remain hysterectomy for the time being. If, however, you have had no children, you may wish to consider the progesterone therapy, but it will be explained to you that there is a risk of cancer recurrence. As long as this happens within the uterus, then you still will have a curable disease. However, there are some women who develop secondary spread from endometrial cancer away from the uterus, for instance in the lungs. When the disease is in the lungs, cure is much less likely, and if you have gone down the route of sparing your fertility to discover that you have gone from having a curable cancer to a potentially incurable one, you would quite rightly feel devastated. These are very difficult choices for women to make and there is no doubting that the care you receive must be highly individualised. The risks, benefits, etc. must all be discussed with you in a clear fashion so that you know what to expect and what not to expect. For those women who undergo conservative therapy using progesterone drugs, re-hysteroscopy and re-sampling will take place on a very regular basis to make sure that if the cancer comes back it is hopefully detected early while it is still in the uterus and preferably at stage I, and therefore, curable by surgery alone.

For those women who are left without a uterus, there has been much publicity around uterine transplantation and a number of groups of researchers (Giuseppe Del Priore and I are two) are involved in research in this area. It is, however, important to say that, to date, this is still highly experimental. Professor Brannstrom in Sweden has successfully performed nine transplants in women and Professor Ozkan in Turkey one. Some of these women have now had successful pregnancy. In the UK, we hope to start this procedure in 2015 depending on funding. We, the authors, personally have little doubt that this type of operation will probably become available in the future, but it is unlikely that a proper programme will develop before 2018, i.e., still some years off and this presupposes that there are successful pregnancies in the experimental series currently underway.

Surgical Procedures Referred to in this Chapter

Investigations:	Hysteroscopy, Dilatation and curettage
	Pipelle biopsy and ultrasound
Surgical treatment:	1. Total abdominal hysterectomy and bilateral salpingoopherectomy (TAH, BSO)

2. Laparoscopic: TLH, BSO,
3. LAVH, BSO
4. TAH, BSO or
5. TLH, BSO or
6. LAVH, BSO and lymph node sampling
7. Radical lymphadenectomy and TAH, BSO
   Omentectomy

All of these procedures can be performed as robotically assisted.

Chapter 9

Vulval Cancer

General Facts

Vulval cancer is a rare cancer and accounts for only 3–5% of all malignancies in the sexual organs of women. It does appear to be getting commoner and does usually affect women who are elderly. Over half of patients are over the age of 70. Having said this, about 15% of patients will be under the age of 40. The cause of vulval cancer is not fully understood, but it is known that most vulval cancers are preceded by a condition called vulval intra-epithelial neoplasia (VIN). VIN is graded into low grade (VIN 1) and high grade (VIN 2 and 3), and thus there is a sliding scale (see Figure 9.1). We also know that many women with VIN 1 will spontaneously revert to normal. This can also happen with VIN 2 and 3, but usually VIN 2 and 3 require treatment before they will go back to normal. We also know that VIN 2 and 3, if left untreated, would appear to have a high (perhaps 90%) chance of developing into vulval cancer, but over an extremely long period of time, probably on average 20–40 years. Unlike a similar condition in the

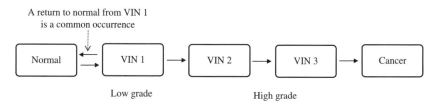

Figure 9.1 Sliding scale of VIN. There is some dispute as to the genesis of VIN 3, but the model that we've shown here pictorially is still helpful in terms of thinking about cancer development.

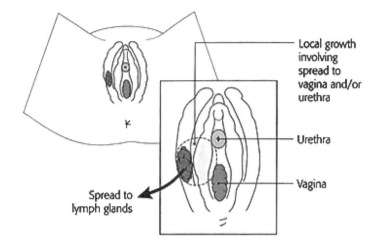

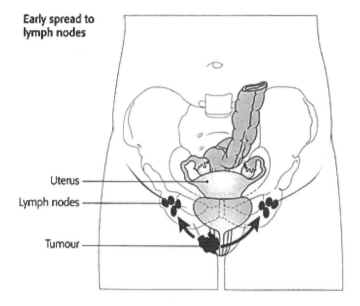

Figure 9.2   Vulval cancer and VIN.

- Many conditions cause vulval itch, or pruritus. Changes in the vulval skin may be noticeable, but this does not necessarily indicate cancer.
- One cause of vulval itching is lichen sclerosis. This is a distressing condition that affects mainly elderly women. Although harmless in itself, women with lichen sclerosis have an increased risk of developing vulval cancer.
- Vulval intra-epithelial neoplasia (VIN for short) is a pre-cancerous condition, and is associated with infection with a virus called HPV. VIN is not a cancer, but it means that the cells are abnormal and have the potential to become cancerous.

Figure 9.2 (*Continue on facing page*)

- It is often not possible to distinguish between a non-cancerous condition and early cancer by appearance alone. VIN and vulval cancer may cause no symptoms, and VIN may appear normal to the naked eye.
- Vulval cancer spreads directly into the tissues next to the vulva, including the vagina, urethra, bladder and anus. Early spread or metastasis occurs though the lymph fluid channels into the lymph glands in the groin, and then to the lymph glands in the pelvis. Less commonly, metastasis occurs through the bloodstream, causing tumours to grow in distant sites such as the lungs and brain.

cervix (CIN, cervical intraepithelial neoplasia), which causes no symptoms, VIN tends to cause itching and discomfort; however, the vast majority of women who have itching and discomfort in the vulva have thrush and do not have VIN. Thrush is very common; VIN is very rare (Figure 9.2).

Other types of skin cancer can sometimes affect the vulva. These are usually dealt with by local removal (see Figure 9.3). VIN is treated either by excising the area as in Figure 9.3, or sometimes with laser treatment. As with all cancers, a staging system, i.e. a system that determines how far the cancer has spread, is used. Table 9.1 shows the various stages of vulval

Table 9.1 FIGO staging of vulval cancer. (Stage 0 is from TNM staging.)

Stage	Criteria
	Primary tumour cannot be assessed.
	No evidence of primary tumour.
0	Carcinoma *in situ* (pre-invasive).
I	Tumour confined to vulva or vulva and perineum, greatest dimension ≤ 2 cm.
IA	Tumour confined to vulva or vulva and perineum, greatest dimension ≤ 2 cm, stromal invasion of ≤ 1.0mm.
IB	Tumour confined to vulva or vulva and perineum, greatest dimension ≤ 2 cm, stromal invasion > 1.0 mm with negative nodes.

(*Continued*)

Table 9.1   (*Continued*)

Stage		Criteria
II		Tumour of any size with extension to adjacent perineal structures (lower third of urethra, lower third of vagina, anus), with negative lymph nodes.
III		Tumour of any size with extension into adjacent perineal structures, with positive inguinofemoral lymph nodes.
IIIA		With 1 lymph node metastasis, any size, or 2 lymph node metastases < 5 mm.
IIIB		With ≥ 2 lymph nodes metastases ≥ 5mm or ≥ 3 lymph node metastases < 5mm.
IIIC		Regional lymph node metastasis with extracapsular spread.
IVA		Tumour invades any of the following: • bladder mucosa • rectal mucosa • upper urethral mucosa or is fixed to bone and/or bilateral regional lymph node metastases.
IVB		Any distant metastasis including pelvic lymph nodes.

cancer. Staging refers to how far the cancer has spread. It allows treatment to be tailored to you, the individual patient, and it allows different hospitals to compare results of different treatments. **The FIGO staging I–IV has no relationship with the 4 cusps A–D.**

Diagnosis

You will probably have noticed either a lump on the outside of your vagina or that you have itching or discomfort, or occasionally bleeding or bad smelling discharge, which will have made you go to your doctor. Your doctor will have examined you and referred you to a gynaecologist. You may have been referred to a colposcopy clinic. (Colposcopy is the microscopic examination of the cervix and vagina and this also can include microscopic examination of the outside of the vagina, i.e. the vulva.) The golden rule with all lumps or ulcers on the vulva is that if there is no infection diagnosed, then your doctor must take a sample to exclude a diagnosis of VIN or vulval cancer. Warts on the vulva are very common, but it is important that, if you have warts, once they have been treated, you are examined to make sure they have gone away. The sample to be taken from the vulva may be done either in the outpatient clinic using local anaesthetic, or it may be done in the operating theatre with you under a general anaesthetic, depending upon the size of sample that one wishes to obtain. Figure 9.3 shows the device used in the outpatient clinic, which removes a very small sample of tissue. If you have had a diagnosis of VIN as stated above, the treatment will be some form of local therapy to remove the area, either by PlasmaJet® laser therapy or by excising it. Sometimes a cream may be used.

Vulval cancer

If the diagnosis is one of cancer, you will have a number of tests performed. These will include checking your blood count to make sure that you are not anaemic, checking your blood salts (urea and electrolytes) and liver function tests. You will have a chest X-ray and since you are likely to require an anaesthetic, you will have an electrocardiograph (ECG). MRI scanning will likely be performed and because these cancers can sometimes spread to the lymph nodes, ultrasound may well be performed of the

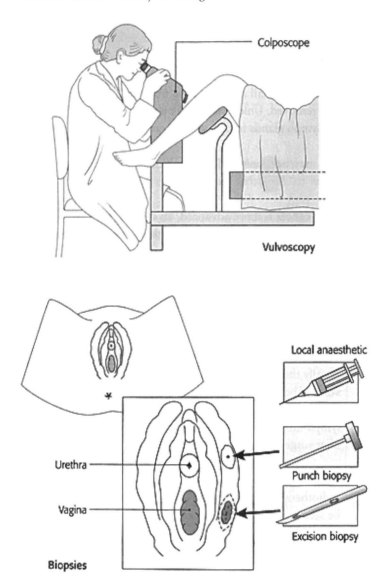

Figure 9.3   Vulval biopsy and treatment of VIN.

- To diagnose vulval intra-epithelial neoplasia (VIN for short), the vulva is examined in a procedure called vulvoscopy. A special microscope called a colposcope is usually used. Vulvoscopy is a painless, outpatient procedure. You will be asked to lie on your back with your legs in supports.
- Dilute acetic acid may be painted onto your vulva to show up any abnormal cells. This is not painful, but may cause mild irritation.

Figure 9.3   *(Continue on facing page)*

- Samples of vulval tissue, called vulval biopsies, may be removed for examination in the laboratory. These are taken either after numbing the area with local anaesthetic, or under a general anaesthetic. Your doctor may take several small circular punch biopsies (tiny circular samples of skin), or remove a larger piece of tissue (called an excision biopsy). You will probably need a few stitches after an excision biopsy, and these will leave a small scar.
- If you have VIN, the abnormal cells may be removed, or sometimes destroyed using a laser. This is usually carried out under general anaesthetic. You will be given painkillers and possibly also a local anaesthetic jelly to use for a few days after treatment.
- After VIN has been diagnosed, you will require regular vulvoscopy. An alternative way of managing this condition is to remove only areas that appear to be progressing towards early cancer. This may save unnecessary surgery.

lymph nodes. Sometimes samples are taken from the lymph nodes using a fine needle. This is also done under local anaesthetic. Sometimes, a CT scan is also done.

The treatment for vulval cancers used to be in the form of very disfiguring surgery, but mercifully, that has now much changed. The drawing shown in Figure 9.4 shows the incisions used if the lymph nodes need to be removed and, as you can see, these leave two almost invisible scars in the groin. Some centres also now offer sentinel node sampling. This involves injection of dyes and radio isotopes to determine if the first drainage node is involved; if it is not, it is very unlikely that any other nodes will be affected. This allows further tailoring of the surgery. With respect to the vulva itself, it partly depends on how big the area is that needs to be removed and its exact position. If it is on one side or the other it is usually possible just to excise the area of the tumour along with an area of normal tissue around it. If the clitoris is not involved with the tumour, great efforts are made to preserve as much normal tissue as possible, so that sexual function will be as normal as possible afterwards. Cosmetically, it is obvious that the less tissue that is removed, the better the result. Having said this, even when a lot of tissue has to be removed, people are usually very surprised at the acceptability of the result once everything has healed up.

For those people who have stage I and stage II, the cure rates are very high. You will be followed up after your operation and seen every 3–4 months for the first couple of years, then probably every six months for

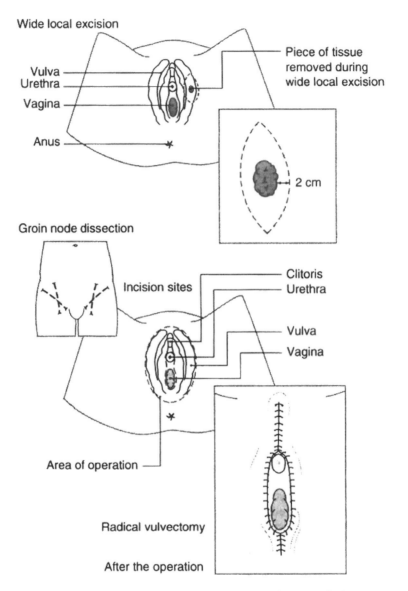

Figure 9.4   Wide local excision, radical vulvectomy and groin node dissection.

- If you have a small vulval cancer, it may be removed under general anaesthetic in a procedure called wide local excision. A small amount of normal surrounding tissue is also removed. Unless the cancer is at a very early stage, the lymph glands in one or both groins are also removed. Sentinel node sampling may be possible.

Figure 9.4 *(Continue on facing page)*

- You may be monitored with vulvoscopy up to four times a year to check that the cancer has not returned.
- If the cancer is more advanced, an operation called partial or complete radical vulvectomy and groin node dissection is usually required. This involves removing the entire vulva and the lymph glands in the groins. Sentinel node sampling may be possible. If necessary, the lower part of the urethra can be removed without affecting bladder function. The skin with the pubic hair is not normally removed.
- The operation is carried out under general anaesthetic, usually though separate cuts in the groins and around the vulva. The skin at the bottom of the vagina is stitched directly to the skin outside of the vulva. Tubes drain lymph fluid from the groin wounds for up to ten days after surgery.
- Depending on the pathology report, you may require radiotherapy after the wounds have healed. You will be seen regularly at the clinic for at least 5–10 years. Penetrative sex is usually, but not always, possible after a radical vulvectomy. If not, reconstructive surgery may be possible at a later date.

the next three years and then probably once a year thereafter until you reach ten years after treatment. Radiotherapy is sometimes required if the lymph nodes are involved and further details with respect to radiotherapy can be found in Chapter 12.

Sexual Function

It is thought that there are four types of women, in terms of orgasmic function: those who achieve deep vaginal orgasms; those who achieve orgasm by superficial clitoral stimulation and external genital stimulation; those who have both; and those who have neither. Operations on the vulva do not have any effect on the type of vaginal orgasm, but if the clitoris is removed and/or the labia minora, it may have an effect on your ability to achieve an external stimulation orgasm. This is part of the reason, as well as the cosmetics of it, for trying to preserve as much tissue as possible. You should discuss this sort of thing with your gynaecologist if you are sexually active, or you may feel more comfortable discussing this with the specialist nurse if you prefer.

Chapter 10

Breast Cancer by Adam Stacey-Clear

Introduction

Breast cancer is the commonest form of cancer in women in Western countries and accounts for 30% of all cancers in women in the UK. In fact, it is the most common cancer in persons in the UK, even though it is rare in men. In 2011, there were 50,285 cases diagnosed in the UK, but the mortality rate has fallen dramatically to the lowest level in 40 years, just 15% of cancer deaths in females. This is due to improvements in diagnosis and treatment. Breast cancer is still the leading cause of death among woman aged between 40 and 50 years of age for all causes put together. It is important to say that 80% of breast cancer occurs in women over the age of 50.

Breast cancer is not one disease as we have now identified many different biological subtypes. This is an incredibly important advance in our understanding of the disease and means that we can offer targeted treatment depending on the tumour biology. This in turn can avoid some of the unpleasant side effects of the other treatments.

Epidemiology

Breast cancer incidence varies depending upon where in the world one lives. It's common in North America and Western Europe, uncommon in Asia and Africa. If women living in Japan (where the incidence of breast cancer is low) move to California, then within a couple of generations, the incidence catches up with the established population. This strongly suggests the role of environmental or possibly dietary factors. Other factors that increase the risk of breast cancer include alcohol, lack of exercise, obesity and increased exposure to the 'oestrogen window'. This refers to women who have an early menarche and a late menopause. Because oestrogens are stored in fat cells, if a woman is very obese at the time of menarche, then the developing breast tissue may receive an unwelcome influence from the high levels of adjacent oestrogen saturated fat cells. Late first pregnancy is of importance because we know that breast feeding in women under the age of 30 can have a protective effect.

There are two well recognised breast cancer genes, namely BRCA1 and BRCA2. If present, then the lifetime risk of developing breast cancer is increased by approximately 40–80%. However, these two genes only account for less than 8% of all the cases diagnosed each year. It is true that family clusters of breast cancer occur without the presence of either of these genes. In these cases, the effect of young age at diagnosis (less than 40) and involvement of first degree relatives may have influence on the risk. It is highly likely that other genes will be discovered that have a less dominant effect, but which nonetheless increase the lifetime risk. The oral contraceptive pill may or may not have a direct influence on breast cancer risk and a great many publications have been produced arguing each way. The oral contraceptive pill appears to greatly reduce the risk of ovarian cancer and endometrial cancer, but its influence on breast cancer may be indirect. That is to say, we know that women who have a late first pregnancy (with breast feeding) lose the protective effect of early pregnancy. Such women may be on the oral contraceptive pill to delay pregnancy, and subsequently may have children much later on. The anxiety behind HRT as a risk factor stemmed from the belief that the prognosis (outlook) for women with breast cancer was worse if they were pregnant when diagnosed. This has now been disproved by comparing outcomes for matched pregnant/non-pregnant women. Of course, administering HRT after breast cancer diagnosis is a very carefully considered option only after close discussion with the oncologist. Long-term administration of HRT for healthy women remains the subject of debate and it may be that a pragmatic view must be taken in each case, perhaps taking into account the family history and even offering increased screening.

In summary, increasing age is the greatest risk factor, carrying the breast cancer gene BRCA1/2 denotes higher risk but actually only accounts for a small proportion of woman getting cancer. HRT, certainly in the first five years of usage, probably confers minimal risk.

Screening

Currently in the UK, breast cancer screening used to start at age 50, but is now being phased in to cover all women aged 47–73. It is undertaken on a three yearly basis by mammography. Mammograms are done by taking X-rays of breast tissue. The breast is compressed between two plates, which can sometimes cause discomfort, particularly if you have small breasts. In North America and other Western European countries, mammogram screening often starts at age 40. In women with a significant family history, and after advice from a genetics councillor, a screening programme starting at a younger age may be advised. In general, the value of mammography in women under 35 is less effective because the breast tissue is denser. Ultrasound screening is of no use whatsoever because it is not reproducible from one year to the next, nor does it provide enough detail. In some circumstances, women with a cluster of family members diagnosed under the age of 40 may be offered MRI (magnetic resonance imaging) screening.

The overall lifetime risk of a woman developing breast cancer, i.e. from age 20–85, is 1 in 12. However, this risk includes those women known to be at increased risk, e.g. genetic abnormality, and therefore the actual risk is probably considerably less. Remember that 80% of all cases occur in women over 50, which is why the screening age range starts shortly before then. Patient surveys show that women overestimate the risk of dying from breast cancer in the next ten years by 22 times and overestimate the benefit of screening by 127 times. It is therefore fair to say that in strict cost–benefit terms, the UK screening programme is ideal. It may be that combining a mammogram with a cervical smear and measurement of blood pressure would result in even more health benefits, but there would be a cost implication.

Some company schemes offer annual mammographic screening from age 40. Mammograms are not dangerous to the normal population and the radiation exposure is the same as six weeks normal background radiation. In other words, we all have a 'mammogram dose' every six weeks and one extra per year is not going to cause any harm.

Figure 10.1 is a drawing of the breast showing the various structures within it. Figure 10.2 shows where breast cancers arise and these very rarely start in breast tissue which is not glandular tissue; in other words,

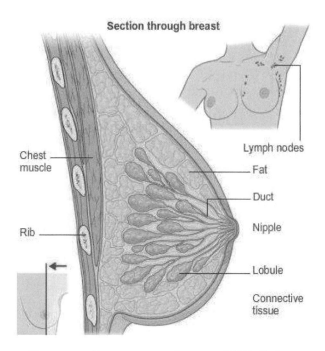

Figure 10.1   Breast anatomy. Courtesy of NHS Choices.

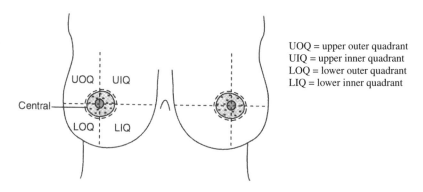

Figure 10.2   Possible sites of tumours.

the tissue that is designed to make milk. Of breast lumps discovered, 90% are benign, but naturally cause a lot of anxiety. The benign lumps include fibro adenoma, simple cysts or benign mastitis infections. In addition, trauma to the breast tissue can result in bruising and damage to the fatty tissue surrounding the normal glandular tissue. This is called traumatic fat necrosis and is commonly found in the inframammary fold where an under wired bra can cause uncomfortable lumpy areas.

However, for the woman who has a breast cancer, this will be staged, i.e. information relating to the size and extent of the tumour is gathered in order to help plan the most up to date treatment. It is important not to confuse stage with grade, the latter being a score allocated by the pathologist and which describes how closely (or not) the cancer cells resemble normal breast gland cells. Tables 10.1 and 10.2 show the staging for breast cancer. The most widely used classification is the tumour-nodes-metastases (TNM classification of breast cancer).

There is also the Union Internationale Contre Cancer (UICC) staging system for breast cancer which incorporates the TNM classification.

Table 10.1   TNM classification of breast cancer.

Tumour Status

T0	No palpable tumour
T1	Tumour 2 cm with no fixation*
T2	Tumour >2 cm but <5 cm with no fixation*
T3	Tumour maximum diameter >5 cm with no fixation*
T4	Tumour of any size with either fixation to chest wall or ulceration of skin

Status of lymph nodes

N0	No palpable axillary nodes
N1a	Palpable nodes not thought to contain tumour
N1b	Palpable nodes thought to contain tumour
N2	Nodes >2 cm or fixed to one another and deep structures
N3	Supraclavicular or infraclavicular node

Distant metastases

M0	No clinically apparent distant metastases
M1	Distant metastases obvious

*For T1-3 'a' indicates no attachment to underlying muscles; 'b' indicates attachment.

Table 10.2   UICC staging system for breast cancer.

UICC stage	TNM classification
I	T1, N0, M0
II	T1, N1, M0; T2, N0-1, M0*
III	Any, T, N2-3, M0; T3, any N, M0; T4 any N, M0
IV	Any T, any N, M1

Many expert groups include T2 tumours in stage 1. The average size of a palpable tumour discovered by a patient is 2 cm, but with screening it is often much smaller.

Breast Self-Examination

Breast self-examination has long been promoted as a way to promote earlier detection of cancers, but as can be seen, if 90% of lumps are benign, then much anxiety is caused by breast examination being done by you. Breast examination and breast awareness are now promoted, which encourage women to be aware of their breasts and if they develop dimpling or flaking of the skin, unusual pain or discomfort, nipple discharge, lumps or thickening that is not cyclical, and any new appearance to their breasts, then they should go to see their doctor. Never feel that you might be wasting the doctor's time, no matter how trivial you might think the problem is. Breast pain (mastalgia) is not usually a serious sign as over 90% of breast cancers are painless.

Once You or Your Doctor Find a Lump

Once this has happened you will be referred to a specialist who will do what's called triple assessment, which will involve taking a history (asking questions), examining you and then using a combination of ultrasound, digital quality mammogram and possibly a needle biopsy. Ideally, these are all done on the same day in what is termed a one stop breast clinic. The needle biopsy will be either a fine needle aspiration of cells (which can be examined immediately) or a core biopsy which removes, under local anaesthetic, a larger tissue samples. From this, the pathologist can often obtain a great deal of information about the tumour biology. Occasionally an MRI scan will be requested, often in younger patients. These techniques allow the diagnosis to be made and the initial stage of the tumour as previously shown in Table 10.1 to be worked out. The treatment which you will be offered depends on putting together all the available information, and only after careful discussion of the results with other members of the multi-disciplinary team. It is very important to remember that if caught at an early stage, then breast cancer is now completely curable.

Management of Early Cancer

The goal of the treatment is to provide the best chance of cure. The idea is to accomplish this with the minimum of surgery, minimum of chemotherapy, minimum of hormone therapy and minimum of radiotherapy; in other words, to give the best cure rate with the fewest side effects. Currently, most women will start their treatment with surgery as this is often required to provide all the pieces of the staging jigsaw, and then move onto some form of either hormone therapy or chemotherapy.

Surgical options for breast include conservative surgery — in other words, where the lump itself is just removed — and this is usually accompanied by sampling the local lymph nodes. This has the advantage of retaining the breast. The other option may require removal of the whole breast. This can mean that radiotherapy is not required to the breast, but may still be required to the armpit. Figures 10.3–10.6 demonstrate these procedures.

The surgical procedure recommended will be based on full discussion with the multi-disciplinary team, and then discussed with you in great detail. Patient informed choice is so essential, supported by the breast care nurse. Any complications likely to occur will be explained in great detail. It is important to state that mastectomy does not improve survival as lumpectomy with radiotherapy is just as effective. Mastectomy is indicated for large tumours (greater than 4 cm) or when it is growing in more than one part of the same breast at the same time (multifocal).

The other issue is what to do about the lymph nodes, since removing these often increases the side effects associated with the surgery. Previously the lymph nodes were usually removed and mostly they were found not to

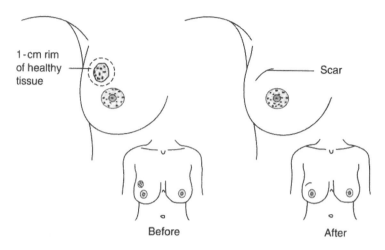

Figure 10.3   Breast lumpectomy/wide local excision.

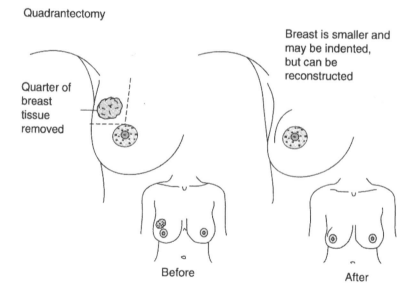

Figure 10.4   Removal of part of the breast.

Simple mastectomy

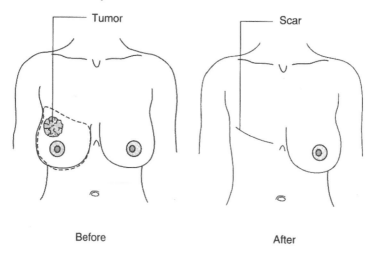

Figure 10.5 Simple mastectomy/removal of the whole breast.

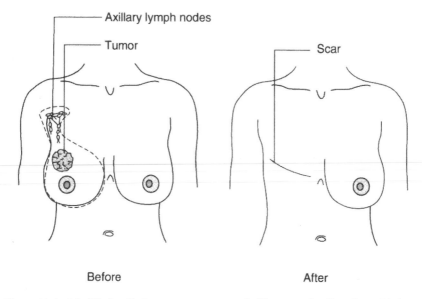

Figure 10.6 Modified radical mastectomy: removal of breast and axillary (armpit) tissue.

have cancer in them, so that in retrospect it seemed to have been the wrong thing to do, to have removed them. Removal of lymph nodes can lead to swelling in the arm and discomfort (lymphoedema). The management of lymphoedema is described on page 151. Much research has gone into trying to identify whether nodes were involved prior to surgery to reduce the number of unnecessary lymph node removals. One of the difficulties is that X-ray techniques such as CT scanning, MRI or ultrasound on their own are not sensitive enough. If the lymph nodes look abnormal on ultrasound scanning, then a fine needle biopsy can be very helpful to see if there are cancer cells present, in which case, the glands can be removed at the time of surgery.

Now the technology of sentinel lymph node biopsy has become available. This allows for removal of just one node to check whether there has been any spread. If there has not, then it is reasonable to assume that the other nodes are not involved with cancer. If the sentinel node is positive, then you can assume that the other nodes are at high risk of involvement and therefore their removal is necessary, subject to confirmation at the breast multidisciplinary team meeting. This has greatly helped to reduce the number of complete lymph node removals (lymphadenenctomies) being undertaken. One of the very difficult things for women to cope with in the past was that they had got bad side effects from the lymph node removal and that it had not been necessary anyway. With careful preoperative selection, it is not necessary to remove all the lymph glands, and even if their removal is necessary, it is possible to minimise the risk of lymphoedema by preserving the arm lymphatic channels and concentrating on those which just drain the breast lymph fluid.

Nowadays, after mastectomy, reconstructive surgery is also possible and there are many different ways of doing this. It may be done at the same time as your initial operation or it may be done later. These are all issues you should discuss with your surgeon or your breast cancer specialist.

Radiotherapy

Most women will have radiotherapy after their surgery if they have had conservative surgery; in other words, the lump only removed and the treatment given is usually delayed by six weeks after surgery. The exact amount and duration of treatment will be explained by the specialist. Radiotherapy can give side effects in the form of nausea, skin rashes and occasional inflammation of the lung. It has, however, been shown to reduce the chances of local recurrence of the disease in breast conserving surgery by a further 60%, over and above the result of surgery alone.

In terms of other treatments, chemotherapy might be used depending on the results of surgery, and this may be followed by endocrine blockade against oestrogen with either Tamoxifen or an aromatase blocker. The latter is not effective unless the patient is post-menopausal, and works by inhibiting oestrogen synthesis in peripheral tissues. Tamoxifen can be given at any age, provided the tumour is oestrogen-sensitive (80% of breast cancers are oestrogen receptor positive). Chemotherapy significantly improves survival in selected patients, being best for women with grade 3 cancers (cells look nothing like normal breast cells), lymph node positive (glands involved), oestrogen-insensitive and Herceptin-positive (a cancer blocking antibody that acts on a growth factor gene found on the surface of 20% of breast cancer cells) cancers. The discovery of Herceptin is one of the most important discoveries in the last ten years. Combined with chemotherapy, it can produce a further 50% reduction in risk of the cancer returning. There is a small risk (2–3%) of minimal heart damage, but special tests will be done to monitor this. Some of the benefit of chemotherapy in women under the age of 50 may be the effect that the chemotherapy has on the ovaries by making the ovaries become menopausal. In other words, it stops them from working and this effect can also be achieved from the use of other drugs designed to stop the ovaries functioning. These are given by injection, either monthly or three monthly (e.g. GnRH analogue). These particular drugs can have an advantage if you are a younger woman looking to have children in the future. The decision to become pregnant after breast cancer treatment should probably be delayed by three years. Chemotherapy may be given to women up to the age of 75, but after this, it may not be effective. Tamoxifen does have side effects, e.g., increased risk of blood clot in the leg veins (venous thromboembolism) and giving or enhancing menopausal symptoms, in other words, flushes and sweats, and very occasionally, endometrial cancer. This has been much hyped up by the press and the risk of endometrial cancer is very rare (one in 1,000 with five years' worth of treatment). However, Tamoxifen reduces the risk of death from breast cancer by 20 to 30%. In other words if your doctor has suggested you take Tamoxifen, you should take it as the advantage would appear to be very high. Recent research trials suggest that the benefits are maximised by taking it for up to ten years. As already indicated, there is no point in taking Tamoxifen if your tumour hasn't got any oestrogen receptors; in other words, if it hasn't got the right factors in the breast to make the Tamoxifen work. Your breast tissue that was removed would be analysed for oestrogen and progesterone receptors, the two common female hormones to help tailor the treatment appropriately.

The other class of drugs, the aromatase inhibitors, have some side effects as well, including joint stiffness, bone thinning (which can be detected with a bone density scan, and then treated) and vaginal dryness. In terms of the problems of chemotherapy you should refer to Chapter 13.

Much has been written with respect to hormone replacement therapy for survivors of breast cancer and this can be a very vexed issue. However, as already stated, it's certainly fair to say that breast cancer is not an absolute counter indication to taking hormone replacement therapy and any decision should be based upon the symptoms that you yourself are suffering. Advice on this will always be given by the breast specialist so that you can make an informed choice.

Management of Advanced Cancer

The goal of the treatment here is unfortunately not to achieve cure, but to give you the best quality of life possible with minimal side effects from the treatment that is suggested. The treatment may incorporate chemotherapy, hormone (endocrine) therapy, surgery and radiotherapy, depending upon where your disease is. If the disease is in the bone, there are good responses from radiotherapy, which can give very good relief of symptoms, the principle symptom of course being pain. Readers are referred to Chapter 13 on pain management. Breast cancer and bone pain, can also be treated with drugs called bisphosphonates, which are very good for controlling the calcium levels in your bloodstream and can be very good for pain associated with secondary cancer in the bone.

Sex and Body Image

While the new approaches to smaller operations, less removal of lymph nodes and better reconstructive surgery have all greatly helped women from a body image and self-esteem point of view, the diagnosis is still shocking. In my experience, women never take things for granted ever again and are keen to have extended surveillance after treatment. There are many support groups and drop in centres where you can meet other women who have been through the same trauma. The breast care nurse will have shown you all these options.

In general terms, Chapter 18 on bereavement is very worthwhile reading because it goes through the range of emotions you will experience in the wake of your diagnosis. Specific issues with respect to sex and body image can often be helped by counselling, psychotherapeutic interventions and complementary techniques such as self-hypnosis, which is described in Chapters 14 and 15.

How Do I Cope With My Diagnosis and Disease

If you have breast cancer that has been detected early and treated where the goal has been to achieve cure, you will be followed up on a regular basis with examinations to check the breast and intermittent blood tests and X-rays. Follow up after breast cancer diagnosis varies depending on local protocols. It is designed to decrease anxiety, not increase it. One of the great difficulties with all cancers is the fear that it will come back, and breast cancer like all other cancers can come back. Unfortunately, slightly differently from many of the pelvic cancers, it can come back after many years. In other words, all is well for many years and then it can reappear. With breast cancer, 75% of recurrences are found by the patient between clinic appointment visits and, therefore, an open access rapid re-referral system is so important. Your GP should always be able to help with this.

Most of the other cancers described in this book, if they have gone for five years are very unlikely to reappear. Readers are referred to Chapter 3. Chapter 19 on spirituality again may make for useful reference.

Useful Addresses

National Institute for Health and Care Excellence (NICE):
https://www.evidence.nhs.uk/topic/breast-cancer
Macmillan Understanding Breast Cancer:

http://www.macmillan.org.uk/Cancerinformation/Cancertypes/Breast/
Breastcancer.aspx
NHS, Causes of Breast Cancer:
http://www.nhs.uk/Conditions/Cancer-of-the-breast-female/Pages/
Causes.aspx
Cancer Research UK:
http://www.cancerresearchuk.org/cancer-help/type/breast-cancer/
Adjuvant! Online, program for estimation of risk and benefits of adjuvant
therapy:
https://www.adjuvantonline.com/index.jsp

Chapter 11

Choriocarcinoma — Gestational Trophoblastic Neoplasia (GTN)

General Facts

This condition describes a whole spectrum of diseases, which include hydatidiform mole, invasive mole, choriocarcinoma and placental site tumour. Up until about 40 years ago, if a diagnosis of choriocarcinoma was made for a patient, the cure rate was sadly very low. Fortunately, this has now radically changed and choriocarcinoma is one of the most curable of gynaecological cancers. Hydatidiform moles are not cancers and invasive moles act somewhat like cancers. As with many other cancers, there is a sliding scale in terms of 'aggressiveness'; hydatidiform mole is a local problem, whereas a choriocarcinoma or placental site tumour can be a disseminated problem — in other words, it can spread through the body. Your chances of being cured with this condition are very high, even if it has spread, either by using surgery or chemotherapy or sometimes radiotherapy. Many women, after treatment for this condition, go on to have children.

Hydatidiform Mole

The incidence of this condition varies depending upon where one lives. In the UK and USA, it occurs in about one to three in every 1,000 pregnancies, but in the Far East, it affects one in 77 pregnancies in some areas. It is also related to the age of the mother. The lowest chance of occurrence is when you become pregnant between 20 and 29 years of age and the highest chance is if you become pregnant when you are under the age of 15 or over the age of 40. The condition does not appear to be related to whether you have had children before, what kind of contraception you have used or if you have had radiotherapy or chemotherapy in the past.

Hydatidiform moles are classified as either complete or partial. The complete type have a higher chance of progressing to an invasive mole or choriocarcinoma than the partial type. If you have a complete mole, you have approximately a 7% chance that you will need chemotherapy, whereas if you have a partial mole, the chance is 3%. The partial mole accounts for approximately 15% of all cases.

All of these conditions are part of an abnormality associated with pregnancy. All of the conditions produce a positive pregnancy test in the blood and usually in urinary tests. Pregnancy tests measure the levels of the hormone beta human chorionic gonadotrophin, beta HCG for short, which is normally produced by the placenta during normal pregnancy. Most pregnancy tests bought in pharmacies give either a positive or a negative result. In hospitals, however, pregnancy tests performed on blood give either a negative result or if positive, give a sliding scale from weakly positive to highly positive. Usually, very early in pregnancy, the test is weakly positive and over the first 12 weeks, it becomes more positive, before subsiding thereafter. In choriocarcinoma, the test in the blood is very strongly positive. Ironically, although the beta HCG levels may be very high, the urine pregnancy test may be negative. The reason that the blood test is strongly positive is because the hormone beta HCG is raised. This is the hormone that causes feelings of nausea and morning sickness in early pregnancy. If you have a hydatidiform mole, you may have exaggerated symptoms, i.e., lots of early morning sickness, etc. in the early part of the pregnancy. In a normal pregnancy, half of the genetic content of the baby comes from the man and half from the woman. The man's half is contained within the sperm and the woman's half within the egg produced in the ovary. Where a complete mole has developed, an empty egg is fertilised by the male sperm and the complete genetic content is male only. There is no baby, no foetus and only an after-birth and a grape-like substance that fills the uterus. In the partial mole, a foetus is present. Instead of there being the normal two sets of chromosomes, there are three sets of chromosomes and the foetus dies usually in the first few weeks of pregnancy.

Usually you will have noticed that your periods have stopped and you felt pregnant, or perhaps there might have been bleeding suggesting a miscarriage. Very occasionally, people see the grape-like things passing from their vagina along with the blood. Sometimes the condition can also cause the blood pressure to be raised and the thyroid gland in the neck to be overactive. Nowadays, the diagnosis is usually made at ultrasound scanning, but sometimes the diagnosis is made following evacuation of the uterus either because of a suspected miscarriage or sometimes because of termination of pregnancy. Because the molar tissue secretes beta HCG, even after you have had an evacuation, the pregnancy test will remain positive and the signs of pregnancy which you may have felt, may well continue. Treatment for a hydatidiform mole is by removing the contents from the uterus. This may have to be done on two occasions to completely empty the uterus and your gynaecologist may do this with the help of an ultrasound machine on your tummy to confirm that the uterus has been emptied (see Figure 11.1).

If you have had a diagnosis of a hydatidiform mole made and then confirmed with evacuation of your uterus, the decision as to whether you need any more treatment is based upon the following:

- Your beta HCG level, which will be measured every 1–2 weeks until it is negative on two occasions. It will be measured every two months for a year and you will be advised to use contraception, other than the combined oral contraceptive pill, for 6–12 months. In addition, physical examination is carried out, including examination of the vagina, cervix and uterus, every three months for a year. You will also have had a chest X-ray which, assuming it is normal, is reassuring.
- If, however, your beta HCG level stops going down or rises, or there was anything detected by way of spread of the molar tissue, then you would be started on chemotherapy immediately.

Gestational Trophoblastic Neoplasia (GTN)

Gestational trophoblastic neoplasia is classified into stage 1, where there is no evidence of disease spread outside the uterus, and stage 2, where there is disease spread outside the uterus. The second type, where there is spread of disease outside of the uterus, is divided into A and B. A is where there

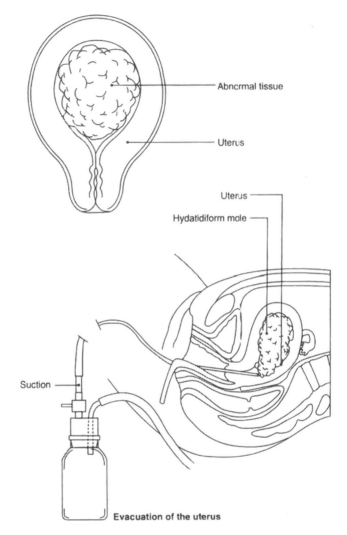

Figure 11.1 Uterine evacuation under ultrasound guidance.

is what is referred to as 'good prognosis metastatic disease' and B is where there is 'poor prognosis metastatic disease'.

The risk of recurrence of gestational trophoblastic neoplasia in people who have no spread outside of the uterus is negligible as the success of treatment is virtually 100%. Where there is 'good prognosis spread outside the uterus', again there is close to 100% success of treatment and where the prognosis is regarded as poor and there is disease outside of the uterus, the success rate still remains high, in the region of 70%. Another way of looking at this is that the chance of the disease recurring if there is no spread outside of the uterus is 2.1%; if there is good prognosis spread outside the uterus, it is 5.4%; and if there is poor prognosis outside the uterus, it is 21%. Where recurrence happens, re-treatment is feasible and for a very small minority of women, further surgery may be required. This combination of treatments makes it very unlikely that women with gestational trophoblastic neoplasia will be anything other than cured of their disease. In addition, the vast majority will retain their fertility.

Section III

General Treatments and Care

Chapter 12

General Concepts of Chemotherapy and Radiotherapy

Chemotherapy can be used in most of the cancers that affect women's gynaecological organs, although the commonest time when chemotherapy is used is for women who have ovarian cancer. There are lots of misconceptions that people have about chemotherapy. First, and most important, is that one often hears people say 'it doesn't work'. This simply is just not true. The difficulty with chemotherapy is in some ways having a picture in your mind's eye of what a cancer looks like and then imagining a drug being poured in, usually via a drip into a vein, and then thinking how that can get rid of cancer. The authors can quite honestly personally testify to having looked inside lots of people's tummies before chemotherapy and after chemotherapy and the difference is truly staggering. Lots and lots of tumour just literally disappears into thin air after chemotherapy.

Currently there are enormous advances taking place in new drug development in the field of chemotherapy. Between the 1970s and 2000, approximately one new drug appeared every five years. Since 2000, there have been five to eight new agents discovered per year! This is influencing the traditional way drugs were evaluated, namely by the randomised controlled trial. This is where two or more groups of patients are randomised (selected by chance) to receive a treatment. The results are then compared over a five to ten year period. This worked well when there was only one new drug every five years, but does not work when there are lots of new drugs. This is where the new science of molecular typing of tumours has come from. The idea is that one grows cells from your tumour and then sees which agent will work in the laboratory before giving it to you. This is similar in idea to what happens when you think you have a urinary tract infection. You go to the doctor and pass urine. The sample is sent to the laboratory where any bacteria in it are grown; they are then tested against different antibiotics to see which ones work. This idea is still in its infancy with chemotherapy but it is partly why you will be asked if it is possible to retain some of the tissue removed from you.

What is true to say about chemotherapy is that it varies in it its effectiveness. Partly this is down to whether the tumour is sensitive to the chemotherapy that is being prescribed and if it is sensitive, how sensitive is it? Some people will make very little response to chemotherapy and some people will make a huge response to chemotherapy. The response of the majority will lie somewhere between these two extremes. The difficulty is that one never knows what response one will make until one has taken the chemotherapy.

In practical terms, chemotherapy usually involves going to the medical day unit or perhaps being admitted to the ward for one day every 1–3 weeks, depending upon what is being given. A drip is put up (see Figure 12.1) and the drug is given through this drip over the course of the day. Various blood tests have to be taken as the chemotherapy progresses to make sure that there are no untoward side effects developing. People worry greatly about the side effects, particularly nausea and vomiting and while these do still occur, they are not nearly as severe as they used to be, partly because the drugs have become more refined, but also because there are newer drugs, which can be given to stop feelings of nausea and vomiting. Probably the biggest worry in terms of side effects is hair loss, which for most is a very disturbing side effect. There are, however, many groups of drugs that do not involve hair loss and for those that do, it is very important to say that hair will grow back after the treatment has finished and often more luxuriantly than it was before. Strangely, some people who have curly hair grow it back straight and some people with straight hair grow back curly hair. This sort of feature is quite unpredictable. What is completely predictable is that the hair will grow back.

Another side effect is that of feeling tired, and there is no doubting that as the treatments progress, people begin to feel much more tired.

Chemotherapy

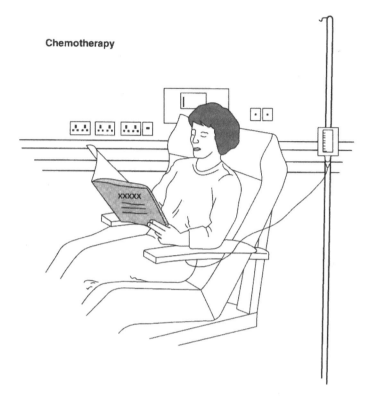

Figure 12.1 Chemotherapy.

One of the authors' own friends who had chemotherapy was able to come around to his house for dinner after his first 'pulse' of chemotherapy. Each time you come in for your dose of chemotherapy, this is referred to as a 'pulse' and as each pulse is given, people tend to feel progressively more tired. The friend, mentioned above, was able to come around for dinner to eat a hearty meal, washed down with a couple of glasses of wine, without feeling in any way unwell.

An unusual side effect can be peripheral neuropathy, which can cause troublesome symptoms including tingling, burning and pain in the limbs including hands and feet. These and the treatments available are discussed on page 151.

Chemotherapy tends to be given in a number of pulses, usually five as a minimum or 12 as a maximum, although this will very much depend upon what drug is being given for what condition. For those of you who have cancer in the vagina or cervix, chemotherapy may be given as treatment alongside radiotherapy and this is to maximise the chances of cure. It fulfils the maxim that you should always hit cancers hard and hit them fast, and hitting a cancer with both radiotherapy and chemotherapy can sometimes be more effective than one of these treatments alone and more effective than surgery.

Radiotherapy can either be used as the main treatment for gynaecological cancers or it can be used as an addition following surgery or chemotherapy. Again, with radiotherapy, it is often difficult to visualise exactly how a tumour can be cured and made to completely disappear, when you feel nothing and see nothing during the treatments, but many tumours are cured.

Radiotherapy involves the use of equipment that delivers a dose of radiation to a specific site. The radiation may be given from an external source (see Figure 12.2) or it may be given internally, with a device placed inside the vagina (see Figure 12.3). Occasionally rods may be placed into the tumour to allow direct access of the radiotherapy into the middle of

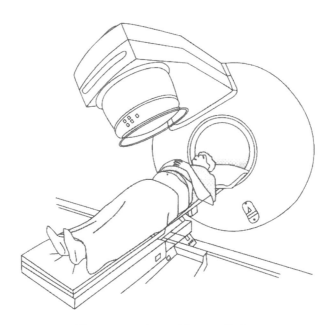

Figure 12.2   External-beam radiation.

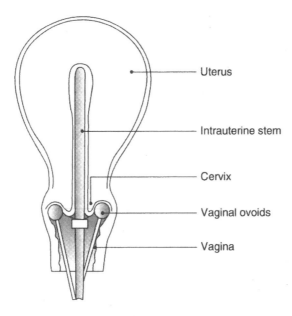

Figure 12.3 Internal radiation (brachytherapy).

the cancer itself. How the radiotherapy is given depends upon where the cancer is, and you should look at the specific chapter, e.g. cervix or vagina, etc. to see the likely method for radiotherapy in your case. In general, radiotherapy is given as a course, where it is given Monday to Friday for a number of weeks. This involves coming to the hospital for a planning meeting, when the whole treatment plan is decided. Thereafter, when you come up to the hospital, you are only there for a few minutes to have the treatment, and then you go home again. You don't actually feel anything at all as the treatment itself is taking place, but over the weeks you may well find that you feel very tired. In addition, you can sometimes get urinary upset with cystitis type symptoms and some bowel symptoms, which can alternate between diarrhoea and constipation and sometimes colicky pain. Very occasionally, you can get pain, tingling and a burning sensation in the skin. All of these things are treatable and some of the treatments are discussed in the chapter on pain management.

Radiotherapy, like surgery, causes long term scarring, which can cause longer term bowel and bladder upset. If you are troubled by symptoms, you should tell your doctor since there are usually effective remedies available (see Chapter 13). It can also result in vaginal narrowing and dryness. Both of these can create difficulty in having sex, including discomfort, pain and bleeding. Graduated dilators and creams can give much relief of symptoms and occasionally minor surgery can help to elongate the vagina.

Chapter 13

Pain Management

Pain and cancer are inextricably linked in all of our minds. I think that probably one of the greatest fears people have when they are given a cancer diagnosis is that it will, at some point, result in them suffering from unbearable pain for which there is no treatment; in general, this is not true and very uncommon. In addition, many people before their diagnosis presume that they cannot have cancer because they have no pain. Ironically, this is one of the greatest misconceptions, since many cancers unfortunately are not discovered until later than they could have been, specifically because they have not caused any pain. This very much applies to problems in the ovary where there are effectively no pain receptors. It is also true that if one feels pain in a leg or an arm or, for instance, in a finger, then the brain is very good at knowing exactly where the pain is, i.e. if the pain is in your right index finger, the problem is likely to be in your right index finger as well. It would be inconceivable that the problem would be in your left ring finger. The same does not apply with pain felt in the internal organs; thus, the ovary tends not to cause pain unless there is bleeding into it and it rapidly expands or if it twists so that its blood supply is cut off, after which the pain will be a diffuse pain, usually arising in the lower abdomen. Pain in the uterus is often felt as lower tummy pain, but can also be felt as lower back pain or upper thigh pain. Even more confusingly, the brain can sometimes mistake pain arising from the right for pain felt on the left and vice versa.

In general, when women come to a gynaecology clinic with pain, the most common cause is that it is arising from the urinary tract, the most common thing being a urinary tract infection or cystitis. The second most common cause is that it is arising from the bowel and often this can be the condition of irritable bowel syndrome, where there are spasms in the bowel often associated with stress. Pain arising from gynaecological organs can be crampy pain associated with periods and bleeding from the uterus. Occasionally, pain can be caused by cysts on the ovary. Two common causes of pain in addition to this are pain caused by infection in the pelvis and pain caused by the condition of endometriosis where the lining of the uterus lies outside the uterus and the pelvis. All of these causes of pain have nothing whatsoever to do with cancer, but can affect the woman who has cancer. In addition to this, cancer itself can cause pain, either because of the damage that it causes to the tissues in your body or because of damage to nerves supplying those tissues, either by applying pressure to the nerves or growing into the nerves. The type of treatment you will need will depend upon the type of pain and, as you can see from what I have written above, the huge number of things that can cause pain mean that the doctor managing your pain is required to ask you a lot of questions and to try to tie in your pain with other symptoms. This may even involve giving people a chart so that they can plot how much pain they get, when they get it and whether it is related to bleeding, urinary function or bowel function.

The rest of this chapter is divided up into 'systems'. By 'systems', I mean whether the pain is related to your bowels or to your urinary tract or to your female organs or, finally, whether it is related to pressure on blood vessels.

Bowel System

Constipation

This is very common, particularly where opiate pain killers have been prescribed, e.g. codeine, morphine or pethidine and can result in severe pain in the back passage (rectum). In addition, if there is a lot of impaction of faeces, then people can get waves of pain as their bowel tries to squeeze out the hard faeces without success. This can be treated using a variety of preparations, such as laxatives e.g., lactulose or senna granules or, failing this, suppositories can be used. For extreme cases, sometimes people have to be admitted to be given enemas to help their bowels move.

Diarrhoea

This can be associated with constipation, where there is diarrhoea, which flows around the constipation. It can also be associated with a tumour pressing on your bowel. Diarrhoea is usually managed with Lomotil or Immodium.

Dry mouth and throat

This can sometimes be a problem during treatments and can cause much discomfort. Use of mouthwashes, sucking on ice cubes or chewing gum can be helpful, and good oral and dental hygiene are important. If you develop oral thrush, nystatin lozenges can be helpful.

Hiccups

These are a distressing thing to suffer from and usually breathing into a paper bag sorts out the problem, but failing this, there are drugs that a doctor can prescribe, e.g. chlorpromazine or amphetamines.

Nausea and vomiting

These are very unpleasant symptoms that can be caused by chemotherapy, radiotherapy and also by opiate pain killers. They are also common symptoms after people have had surgery. There are now, however, extremely good drugs available, for instance, ondansetron or promethazine, which can help with this.

Urinary Tract Problems

Involvement of the urinary tract can cause pain in the lower part of the tummy. It can also cause pain in the small of the back and in the groin. This pain can range from a dull ache to severe 'colicky' type pain. The commonest cause of pain is cystitis, which can be caused by infection, and is easily treated with antibiotics. In addition, cystitis can be caused by radiation, and anti-inflammatory drugs can be helpful with this type of pain. Occasionally pain can be caused by blockage of the ureters (these are the tubes that run between your kidney and bladder) and this can usually

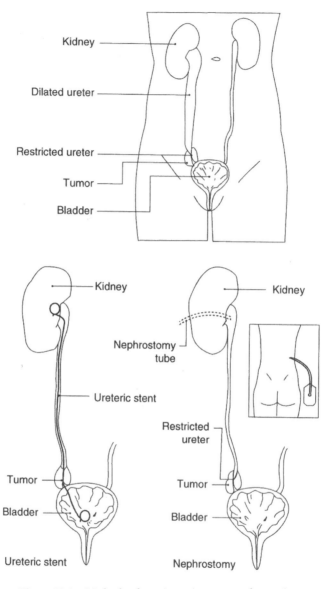

Figure 13.1   Methods of treating urinary tract obstruction.

be relieved by passing a plastic tube down the blocked ureter. This can, either, be inserted in the X-ray department and is known as an antegrade stent, or it can be inserted in the operating theatre via a cystoscope, when it is known as a retrograde stent (see Figure 13.1). It is very important to recognise urinary tract infections, since occasionally this can also cause infection in the kidney (pyelonephritis). Usually if this develops, you would be required to be admitted to the hospital for intravenous antibiotics, through a drip.

Radiotherapy can sometimes cause pain because of tissue scarring and, in addition, a burning pain can be felt in the skin. This can usually be helped by 1% hydrocortisone cream or local anaesthetic cream.

Chemotherapy can cause pain and there is a condition called 'peripheral neuropathy'. This is where there is tingling and numbness in the fingers and toes. This almost always gets better over time, but can be much helped by drug therapy. In addition, chemotherapy can cause inflammation in the mouth and the throat, gullet and stomach, and all of these can be helped by various lozenges, drinks, etc.

Lymphoedema

This is a troublesome condition that occurs when the lymph fluid leaks out of the blood vessels and causes uncomfortable swelling. Lymph fluid is normally collected in channels called lymphatic channels and is transferred back into the bloodstream. After removal of lymph nodes, coupled often with radiotherapy, there is damage to the lymphatic channels and they are no longer able to transfer the lymph fluid back into the bloodstream. The effect of the lymph being unable to get back into the bloodstream is to cause localised swelling. Unfortunately, because of the localised swelling, the swollen area is prone to low grade infections. Sometimes your doctor will give you low dose antibiotics to treat this and will almost certainly suggest certain types of bandaging, and may occasionally offer intermittent pressure boots (see Figure 13.2). They will also suggest that you should elevate the affected area. The elevation encourages the fluid to track back into the bloodstream.

Painkillers

These are also known as analgesic drugs. There is a huge number of drugs that can relieve pain. These have different ways of working. Some of them are anti-inflammatory and some of them are opiate-type drugs. The drug that will be selected for you will be appropriate to your pain. It is important

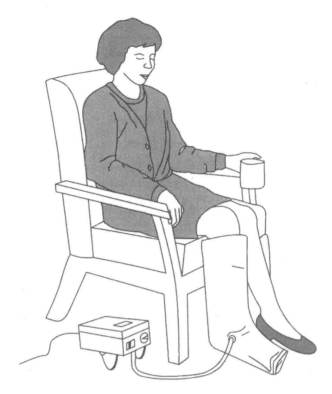

Figure 13.2   An intermittent positive pressure boot for reducing lymph volume.

to say, that amongst this wide variety, these drugs come in differing strengths and clearly your doctor will want to discover what the best drug and best strength is for you. This may change over time, requiring changes of drugs and changes in strengths of drugs. In addition to pain killers, antidepressants can also be used for getting rid of pain. Often people are worried about taking these because they feel that the drug has been given as an antidepressant. In fact, when antidepressants are given as pain killers, they are given in a dose that would not have any effect on depression. They do, however, have an effect on the nerves which are transmitting the pain and this is how they work. Steroids can also be beneficial, since they reduce inflammation and swelling. Chapter 14 on complementary therapies deals exhaustively with complementary approaches to pain. You may, if you are getting problems with pain, find that you are referred to a chronic pain specialist or the palliative care specialist. Both of these groups of specialists are highly experienced in managing pain symptoms.

It is vitally important that you do tell your doctor or specialist nurse if you are suffering from pain, because it is highly likely that they will be able to help your pain by one route or another. In my own experience, it is very rare to find patients with gynaecological cancer in pain for which we have no treatment.

Chapter 14

Complementary Therapies

This chapter discusses the pros and cons of various treatments. It has been written by one of the authors (JRS) and is therefore written in the first person. It is divided into separate sections on hypnotherapy, acupuncture, homeopathy, meditation, spiritual healing and Reike. In addition, there is a section on psychotherapy and counselling. This chapter is designed to give an overview and following this, there are further chapters on hypnotherapy (Chapter 15), nutrition (Chapter 16) and cardiac synchronicity (Chapter 17).

I have not discussed diet in this chapter, because it is fulsomely described by Nigel Denby in Chapter 16. My only comment is that most people know the value of a good balanced healthy diet, with a mixture of food types. There is a great emphasis in the lay press on eating one's way to being disease-free, even potentially not taking proper treatments, and this is nonsense. It is, however, true that one can eat one's way to ill health, while unfortunately, a good diet does not wholly protect one from ill health.

There is certainly no evidence that meat avoidance protects against cancer and in the time around your operation where blood may be lost, red meat can be very beneficial: a steak is equivalent to three iron tablets and better for you.

Hypnotherapy

This technique was originally described by the French physician Mesmer, hence the other name for the hypnotic state, 'mesmerism'. Since its discovery

nearly 200 years ago, it has always remained on the fringes of medical practice. It has undoubtedly gained a variable reputation, partly down to the
antics of stage hypnotists. While there is no doubting the entertainment
properties of the technique, these have overshadowed and undermined the
potential of hypnosis for treatment of a wide variety of conditions. I myself
have taught many patients the ability to self-hypnotise, thus allowing treatment of phobias (e.g. needles, flying, etc.), inability to sleep, wound pain,
menopausal flushes and many other things. The other problem for hypnosis
in terms of acceptance within the medical profession is a lack of research
data to support it, although this is now improving. When I was practicing
in Glasgow, I used to teach self-hypnosis for vaginal pain following child-
birth. At first I wasn't sure how successful this was, until husbands started
bringing me bottles of whisky and boxes of cigars! This may not have been
scientific evidence, but I found it reasonably convincing that I was doing
some good. Hypnosis also has the benefit that for those that it does not help
it rarely does harm. I regularly hypnotise myself, particularly if I can't sleep
or before lectures to big audiences, where it gives me a feeling of calm before
'facing the crowd'. Most of us require three to four sessions to learn the
technique, the first lasting an hour and the others 30 minutes.

The other great fear generated by stage hypnotists is that the technique
allows others to enter into the deeper private parts of your mind and
somehow to gain control over you. In general, no hypnotist can make
people do that which they have no desire to do. There is no doubting that
hypnosis is a powerful tool and that it needs to be done by someone who
you know and trust, either a trained hypnotherapist, doctor, dentist, psychologist or yourself.

In Glasgow in the 1980s, there was a famous stage hypnotist, Robert
Halpern, who during his show appeared to gain complete control of about
50 people in an audience of 1,500 and make these poor unfortunates do all
sorts of ridiculous and entertaining things. Many of my patients who had
seen this show used to ask how I could possibly say that hypnosis did not
give enormous power to the hypnotist. Having seen the show myself I could
tell them that it started by Halpern using a well-recognised method for
testing people's capacity for hypnosis (in general, most people are hypno-
tisable, lack of concentration, cynicism and old age being the main factors
stopping it working). He used a technique where he asked the audience to

clasp their hands together. He then told them that their hands would get tighter and tighter together as he counted from one to ten. With this a high proportion of his audience showed the start of the hypnotic response, but only a few (50 out of 1,500) followed through to the point where they could no longer release their hands. This group of fifty were then invited onto the stage if they wanted their hands released which, of course, they weren't until the end of the show! The group on the stage were then induced into full trance state. The remaining 1,450 people had consciously withdrawn from the hypnotic process. It is reasonable to presume that there will always be a few exhibitionists in every audience!

How does hypnosis work? Nobody knows exactly how it works, but it appears to be a method of allowing access to and control over one's subconscious and deep subconscious. The conscious means that of which we are aware. The subconscious is the activity bubbling away below the surface that we usually only experience in dreams and under the influence of certain drugs. The deep subconscious is that part of the brain controlling things like heartbeat, breathing and other bodily functions that in general we do not 'thinkingly' control. Normally, our conscious self cannot gain entry to or control over our subconscious or deep subconscious. There are exceptions to this: for example, you breathe without thinking but can, if you wish, hold your breath. You cannot, however, control your own heart-rate. Hypnosis allows access to this part of the brain. Examples of this would be that under self-hypnosis you can alter your pulse at will, or a dentist hypnotising you before tooth extraction can stop you salivating and bleeding from the socket. I myself have carried out a number of surgical procedures without anaesthetic under hypnosis with the patient feeling nothing. Figure 14.1 shows a schematic representation of how hypnosis works, allowing access of the conscious to the deeper part of the mind.

I myself select patients who I believe may be suitable candidates for hypnotherapy on the basis of their age, strength of personality and apparent capacity for concentration. Much at odds with what you might think, the best candidates are usually from childhood to middle age and the stronger the personality, the better. If you are an older patient, you may have got to a cynical stage in life making you a poor candidate. None of these criteria are hard and fast and certainly there is little to lose and much to gain by trying.

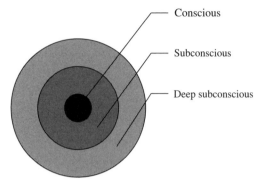

Figure 14.1   Schematic representation of the mind.

It is possible to use the Halpern technique of hand clasping to assess your hypnotisability. Another method is to tell you to close your eyes and that there is a large weight on top of your head and it is getting heavier as I count to ten. I then observe to see if your head starts to nod. In general, it is better to go straight to trying to hypnotise you.

Most people want to know what it will feel like when they are hypnotised. This is not something that one can easily describe. It does however feel slightly 'other worldly', a bit like the 'removed' feeling one gets after taking a sleep-inducing drug. It taps into that place where one is neither awake nor asleep. When you are hypnotised you can talk, hear everything that is going on around you and you can wake up whenever you want, although most people usually don't want to! I always tell people if they feel an itch, or feel uncomfortable, they can move about, scratch themselves or whatever.

Those patients wishing to go ahead are brought back to a clinic where an hour will have been allotted for the first visit, and probably half an hour for each subsequent visit. You will be asked to sit in an easy chair or lie on a couch and firstly to do some gentle breathing exercises. These comprise imagining that there is a candle in front of you. If you are somebody who breathes through your nose, you will be asked to breathe in through your nose and out through your mouth. If you are a mouth breather, you will be asked to breathe in and out through your mouth. The breath out, whichever way you breathe, will last to the count of ten seconds and should be done as if you were slowly blowing out a candle. Doing this for one or two minutes is always very relaxing. You will then be asked to tense various muscle groups and let them relax. I usually start with toes and tell people to tense their toes and relax. Then I ask them to tense their calf muscles and relax, tense their thigh muscles and relax, tense their abdominal muscles and relax. By this time you can feel yourself sinking into the bed. We finish with you tensing the chest muscles and relaxing them, lifting your shoulders and letting them relax and finally screwing up your face and letting it relax.

I then ask you to concentrate on a point which is above and just behind you, enough to make a slight strain on the eyes. I then tell you I am going to count to ten and as I do so, you will feel your eye lids getting heavier and heavier, to the point where you will have to let them close. You should continue to breathe like you are blowing out the candle. As I count to ten, I am watching your eyelids, which usually start to flicker and then close. This is usually an irresistible feeling, quite pleasant and not to be resisted.

I then ask you to imagine that you are on top of a hill, the hill is covered in beautiful lush grass, and you can smell the grass. In Scotland, I used to suggest heather. Overhead is a bright blue sky with the sun shining and a light breeze cooling your face. At the bottom of the hill is a brook, which you can hear babbling in the distance. I am going to count to ten and you are going to walk down the hill. As you do so, you will go deeper and deeper into the hypnotic state. I then count to ten: one, two, three, four, five, you are now half way down the hill and feeling more and more deeply asleep, more and more relaxed, six, seven, eight, nine and ten. Now you are at the bottom of the hill and feeling beautifully relaxed. This process of going down the hill can be repeated two or three times depending upon the patient. I always look for the various signs that it is going well: breathing changes from the chest moving up and down to your tummy moving instead. Occasionally I may think that the patient is just pretending so as not to hurt my feelings; if this is the case, we start again using a different technique.

There are many ways of inducing a hypnotic trance; all, however, utilise similar techniques to those described above. Others include walking down a beach, or counting out loud backwards from one hundred by subtracting three, i.e. 100, 97, 94, etc. Once you are in a deep trance, various approaches can be taken depending upon the initial complaint and the goal of the therapy.

In offering hypnotherapy to patients, I have used it for relief of wound pain, relief of tummy and groin pain, relief of menopausal symptoms in women unable to take hormone replacement therapy, management of needle phobia and as a replacement for general anaesthetic. I have also used it as a confidence builder. Its use as an alternative to general anaesthesia is in general not warranted, since it is extremely time consuming to get a subject to this level of confidence in the technique.

At the end of the hypnotic session you will be taught how to pre-program yourself so you can get into the trance more quickly the next time. I use a process where I press my thumb against my index finger and count one, then on my middle finger and count two, then on my ring finger and count three, then on my pinkie and count four on the inner surface and five on the outer. By doing this, in the future, I induce the same trance in about ten seconds! You will then be told that in the future, you cannot be hypnotised by anybody other than a doctor, a dentist, a psychologist or somebody you know and trust including yourself. This will mean you can go and watch Halpern and the like with complete impunity!

You will then be told that when you wake up you will feel beautifully relaxed and refreshed and that you should count back from five to one in your head and slowly come back awake. This you will duly do, usually with some reluctance since the feeling is so good!

I will illustrate some of the uses from my own experience. Many years ago, I went to a respected hypnotherapist (Shaun Hammond, author of the next chapter) because I smoked twenty cigarettes per day, I was asthmatic, and I was two stones overweight. I was hypnotised and once in a trance, Shaun utilised a schemata derived from Buddhist thinking. In this, you are asked which you see as the most important part of you: your face, your chest, your gut or your groin. These relate to your chakras. We all often describe people as operating on a gut level, or having a big heart or being driven by their groin! For me, my dominant chakra is in my chest. He taught me to imagine my chest opening up like a flower. Once open, it was bathed in bright light and my asthmatic lungs washed with pure water! After this, I was asked to let the power in my chest flow out of it like a fountain. Once I could feel this, I was asked to close the flower down and to make this newly recognised power flow through my arms down to my fingertips. Following this, I was asked to describe where I most liked to smoke. I described the terrace in front of my family's house on one of the islands off the west coast of Scotland (Bute). From there I was taken to a room, my room 101. In it, there was a television and a door. I was in the television and in the room. The 'me' in the television was me 20 years later. By this time, I had developed bronchitis and couldn't breathe without an oxygen mask and I was wracked with terrible coughing fits. Shaun gave me a choice either to be in the television or to walk through a door which had just opened. Through the door was the fresh air and sunshine of Bute and being a non-smoker. I started to walk to the door but hesitated at the door, the hypnotherapist asked what I wanted to do? Be in Room 101 as a smoker or in the fresh air as a non-smoker; this time I walked through the door and haven't smoked a cigarette in 25 years. I did not put on weight; in fact, I lost two stones. This and saying no to cigarettes proved very easy. At any time I was tempted to over eat or smoke, I would self-hypnotise and, utilising the power of the chest chakra, I would have no difficulty in what I can only describe as (psychologically) pushing away the offending item.

I do a lot of lecturing to medical students, other doctors and patient groups. Before lectures where there is a big audience, there are few who will not admit to feelings of nervousness. When I am sitting at the front of the audience just a few minutes before going to the podium I will self-hypnotise using the quick induction technique described above. I then imagine the power in my chest chakra flowing through my arms into my hands and into my fingers. I instantly feel relaxed and tell myself that the lecture will go well. I then count back from five to one and feel relaxed and confident!

I have illustrated above how you can be hypnotised and some of its uses. There are innumerable problems that it can be used for. One of the biggest difficulties is in finding a respectable practitioner, but personal recommendation or using a member of the Society of Medical and Dental Hypnotherapists or a psychologist is usually a route to being safely taught how to self-hypnotise.

Acupuncture/Shiatsu

This is an ancient form of Chinese medicine based on meridians. There are two schools of practice, one the traditional Chinese method, which sees the body in holistic terms. The needles may be heated and herbs applied to the top of the needles. Traditionally, these needles were reused and, as you can imagine with the risks of Hepatitis B, and HIV, strict sterilisation is now needed if needles are to be reused. Many non-Chinese doctors, nurses and physiotherapists now use acupuncture usually as a form of pain relief. Modern medicine does not wholly understand how the acupuncture needle points work.

Shiatsu and acupuncture rely on the same points in the body. These theories arose in the Far East in Japan and China and are based on a theory of 'energy lines' in the body. These can be affected either by pressure or the use of needles. Shiatsu is a form of massage utilising these meridians by pressure; acupuncture involves the insertion of needles.

Acupuncture has become very popular for pain relief both with doctors practicing Chinese medicine and chronic pain specialists. In the UK and USA, many pain specialists who usually have started their training as specialists in anaesthesia have learnt acupuncture and incorporated this into their pain relief practice. I know that two of my own colleagues, one a pain specialist and the other a gynaecologist, use it regularly to help their patients with pain. The needle is placed at a site distant from where the pain is according to the meridian principle, e.g. pain in the upper part of the mouth is relieved by a needle in the ear lobe.

There is no doubt that many patients have gained great relief through this method, as well as enhanced feelings of wellbeing. We do know that the needles release the body's endorphins. These are opiate-like substances produced in all of us, which are not dissimilar in chemical structure to the opiate drugs, such as morphine, which is used as a painkiller. What is not understood is how pressure in one place induces pain relief in a distant part of the body. Another use is the relief of nausea from pressure over the wrist. Useful addresses and information are available on page 227.

Homeopathy

This is a very popular form of alternative therapy, which utilises a system of medicines that are derived from plants, minerals and animal products. In scientific terms, the theory behind homeopathy is counter-intuitive. The homeopathist, who may well be a qualified doctor, will take your history and take into account your physical needs and your emotional needs. They will then identify a medicament that if given to a healthy person would give them your symptoms. The remedy is then diluted down, up to nine times. The more the dilution, the stronger the expected effect; this is the part that the rationalist has to find counter-intuitive. Notwithstanding that we don't understand how it works, many patients seem to derive great benefit from these treatments. In the medical journals, the debate continues much as it has for the last 200 years as to the effectiveness of these treatments. For my money, if something has been around for that amount of time, there must be something in it, even if we don't understand it! Recently, there has been a much greater effort on the part of the homeopathic community to subject their medications to trials, much as standard drugs are. These suggest that some remedies do reliably produce the desired effect! In the UK, there are two homeopathic hospitals, one in London and one in Glasgow.

Alexander Technique

I include mention of this technique for completeness. It is an approach to the way we stand, hold ourselves, walk and sit. It is of great benefit to those suffering from neck and joint pain, breathing disorders and stress-related disorders. It is particularly popular with musicians, especially violinists, who by nature of their job, place their bodies in unnatural positions. It also makes people usually gain an inch or two in height once they have learnt the technique — maybe I should try it myself — I could certainly do with gaining vertical inches rather than horizontal ones!

Massage, Reflexology, Meditation, Yoga, Spiritual Healing

The placing of all of these different techniques under one banner is not intended as any insult or diminution in any particular one. They are, however, all a bit like a Venn diagram, (see Figure 14.2). I don't know if you remember them from school maths.

Massage is a system of stroking, kneading and pressing different areas of the body to relieve stresses and strains; it is particularly good for muscle and joint pains. I doubt if there is anybody who doesn't feel better after massage. Reflexology again originated in the Far East and is a form of

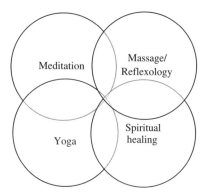

Figure 14.2   Venn diagram.

foot/hand massage, again relying on meridians for an effect distant from the foot.

To my mind, meditation, self-hypnosis and the mental side of yoga are all one and the same thing. There are various exercises whereby one can gain access to the subconscious, the inner self. Chapter 19 on spiritual aspects also deals with this. Yoga is very popular. It was invented in India and is a method of harmonising mind, body and emotions, using posture, breathing, movement and meditation to achieve feelings of wellbeing.

Psychotherapy

There are a number of different approaches to psychology. Historically, psychology started at the beginning of the 20th century with Freud. CG Jung (Figure 14.3) was originally a 'disciple' of Freud before breaking with him and developing his own approaches. These have continued to be developed and are currently taught at many places, amongst them the Jungian Institute at Kusnacht on the shores of the Zurichsee (Figure 14.4). Adler followed with a different approach again. Modern psychologists will have learnt a medley of these approaches. There is also a 'crossover' between orthodox psychotherapists and some complementary therapists who have also been trained in aspects of psychotherapy. The British Society of Psychotherapists website is extremely useful for further information.

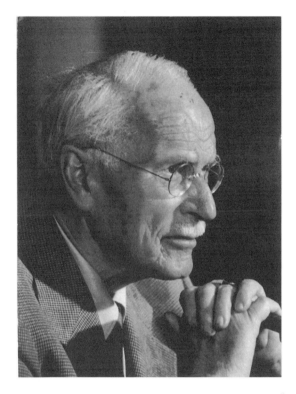

Figure 14.3 CG Jung.

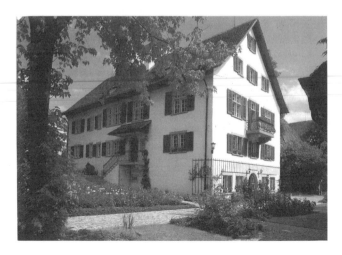

Figure 14.4 Jungian Institute.

A form of psychotherapy known as logotherapy has also become popular. This was invented by Dr Vicktor Frankl, a doctor who was imprisoned in Auschwitz concentration camp during the Second World War and survived. His principal observation was that the few who survived the death camp had a unifying feature, namely a belief that they were here for a purpose. Logotherapy is a psychological method of helping patients discover this side of themselves.

Counselling

There is a plethora of counselling services available to people these days. How much a person wants to talk about their condition varies from one individual to another. To my mind, the meeting together of groups who have suffered similarly, perhaps with a counselling facilitator, seems to help many. I have no doubt that many people are genuinely helped by counsellors, but I also have no doubt that we live in an age where we are on the opposite swing of the pendulum from the 'stiff upper lip' approach, where we were encouraged to not talk about anything. We have now arrived at perhaps a time of over intense 'navel-gazing' and a compulsion to talk about our problems, which does not suit everyone. I'm sure that somewhere in between, which is tailored to the individual, is best!

As you will detect, of the complementary therapies discussed, the only one which I have personally practiced is hypnotherapy. I have developed a network of colleagues to whom I refer to for the other treatments. What people select is largely a matter of their personal preference, though some don't want any of these things, but most will find that at least one appeals to them.

Chapter 15

Hypnotherapy by Shaun Hammond

Editorial note from JRS: I have referred to Shaun since 1988. At the time, I was running a hypnotherapy clinic at St. Mary's Hospital, London and Shaun was too. When I got stuck, I took to referring to Shaun who always seemed to have the answer. When I became a Consultant, I no longer had time to practice hypnotherapy and have since then worked closely with Shaun. His chapter shows great discernment in the art and practice of hypnotherapy and a more sophisticated approach than my own, which I have already described to you in the previous chapter.

Hypnotherapy

If you have just received a cancer diagnosis, there are so many thoughts that must be going through your mind. Not only do you have to deal with the medical interventions that are available to you, but also, you may be interested in taking on a complementary approach in order to broaden your possibilities for self-healing and coming to terms with your diagnosis.

There is such an array of complementary therapies available to you and hypnotherapy is one of them. In writing this chapter, I wish to offer you a broad outline of the skills which can be learnt through hypnotherapy and some of the techniques which are available to you. Naturally hypnotherapists work in many different ways, and so this is just an overview of some of the techniques available to you, and the ones which I use myself on my patients. I feel it is also important to go into some detail about what hypnosis is, and help to de-mystify it as much as possible, as it remains a mysterious and unfathomable form of therapy in many peoples' eyes. Likewise, I have gone into some detail about the subconscious and how it is an amazing asset to you.

Although hypnosis is becoming more recognised, there are still many people who are both fearful and suspicious of it. There is often a lack of comprehension in the difference between stage hypnosis and therapeutic hypnosis. It has to be said that the fear of hypnosis comes from the public seeing the many 'spectacles' of stage hypnosis where participants are apparently made to say and do ridiculous things. There is a whole psychology behind these shows, which I do not have time to go into; however, let me say that it is the deep wish within the participant to do as the hypnotist says which allows them to behave in such strange ways. Also, while the participant is in a relaxed state, their defence mechanisms are less pronounced and so the embarrassment and maybe humiliation of saying and doing strange acts is less marked. So it comes as no surprise that the general public often has an innate fear of hypnosis.

Now, let's look at what hypnosis actually is! It is quite difficult to explain the phenomenon of hypnosis. In simplest terms, it is a natural form of relaxation that can be induced through suggestions given by a hypnotist, or it can be self-induced when a person has learnt how to use the skills to achieve it. While in relaxation, it allows the participant to turn their attention away from their outer awareness and go into their inner thoughts, memories, wisdom and inner knowledge. The suggestion of the hypnotist allows the person to do this in a simple and easy manner. It is at this point that I should mention the relationship between the relaxed state of hypnosis and the levels of consciousness within every individual. Our 'outer awareness' is what we are experiencing at any given moment in time, our 'inner awareness' is everything else we experience (i.e., memories, intuition, automatic responses and the whole functioning within our body). This is what we call our subconscious mind. It can be said there are two layers within the subconscious. The outer layer, which is concerned with our memories, intuition, visions and emotions, and a deeper inner layer, which is about the functioning of our physical body in aspects, such as breathing, our heartbeat and the ability to talk without thinking, and in fact every communication and connection within our physical body. While relaxing in hypnosis, it allows us to go deeper into our awareness at different levels, so this is a state of being that can be implemented as a therapeutic tool in helping people with both emotional and physical difficulties in their lives.

From now onwards, I'm going to use the word hypnotherapist as opposed to hypnotist. This is because generally speaking, a hypnotist is merely a person who has the ability to hypnotise someone, whereas a hypnotherapist is someone who uses hypnosis as part of their therapeutic skills. To clarify the naturalness of the relaxation within hypnosis, it can be said that light hypnosis is an everyday event that we experience at some time. When you are reading a book and your mind is captivated by it, you are in a state of light hypnosis, because your attention leaves your outer awareness and is absorbed by the inner world of the book that you are reading. Another example would be when you are remembering something, especially when this is in detail. Once again your attention shifts from the outer world to your inner world of experiences, visions and memories. What is actually happening is that you are leaving your outer consciousness and going inwards to the inner world of your subconscious mind. The deeper and more vivid these experiences are, the deeper you are in your subconscious mind. Perhaps a more surprising example is when you are driving from A to B and you know the journey so well, you are 'on automatic pilot' in getting to your destination. In this situation, you are accessing the memories of your experience of the journey and automatic reactions within yourself in order to complete it. Sometimes, as we all remember, there are whole parts of the journey we might have forgotten, yet we have arrived at our destination safely. In this case, we have been driving almost completely from a subconscious perspective.

You may be wondering by now how therapeutic hypnosis can be associated with the above examples. It is simply a way of showing you that a hypnotic state is a method of going inside ourselves to help us find our inner resources, memories, gifts, wisdom, knowledge and self-healing and also the ability to trust our automatic responses and reflexes within ourselves. Without our subconscious mind, we would not be able to function in any way at all, and I often describe it as being 'the perfect co-worker inside us', to help us understand and unravel our problems, both physically and emotionally. It is also our best co-worker because its function is to regulate everything in as balanced a fashion as possible in order that we can function in our lives.

One of the major difficulties in dealing with cancer is the fact that patients often feel completely out of control of their situation. Often their diagnosis is a complete surprise, and so there is the initial shock to have to deal with, as well as how they feel their life is going to unravel from that point on. There is often a sense that something is taking them over and there is nothing they can do about it. If it hasn't already happened, an operation and chemotherapy/radiotherapy may follow on. In other words, they often feel powerless and totally out of control. Not only do they have to deal with how they feel about themselves, but also how to function with family and friends around them, so this puts on added pressure to the difficult feelings they are experiencing. As has already been mentioned, hypnosis allows the patient to gain access to all the positive aspects of the subconscious mind, as well as having the knowledge of how to relax in a simple way. Just the ability to relax can often help the patient sort through their various feelings and emotions. This is where self-hypnosis (i.e. the ability to hypnotise oneself) is such an important element within the therapy. When patients realise they can hypnotise themselves without the hypnotherapist being there, it brings a feeling of greater confidence to them, and they realise that they can work on their emotions and physical feelings in between sessions. Also, it means that the patient isn't solely dependent on the hypnotherapy session itself. They can manage their trance states and work on various skills and tools which have been shown to them by their therapist, and in turn bring ideas, thoughts and new realisations to the following therapy sessions. It allows the cancer patient to feel more independent and also being more in control of their self-healing.

It is also important for the cancer patient to find a therapist who understands a similar belief system, i.e., the way they think. This means the hypnotherapist really listens carefully to what the patient is saying, and can pick out the best way forward for the patient, according to what is being said. Some patients have a deep spiritual understanding and how this may be important to them, whether religion has a large part to play, or if the patient is pragmatic in approach. Basically this means that the hypnotherapist is tuning in to the patient correctly and this will bring about a better rapport all around, i.e., they are speaking the same language. The result is that the cancer patient will feel much more understood, and in turn, this often allows the patient to express feelings more openly and deeply.

Preconditioning (i.e., clarifying what hypnotherapy is) the patient to the naturalness of hypnosis is very important as well, because it allows them to relax before the hypnotic experience begins. One of the most important messages that I say to patients is that whatever they feel or experience while in the trance state is always 100% correct! In other words, if they don't see what I'm suggesting they visualise, or their mind goes off in a different direction to what I am suggesting, that it is perfectly okay. This is because the suggestions that I'm giving will still enter the subconscious anyway. Sometimes I explain it like this: 'Imagine there is a buffet in front of you, and you can choose whatever you want to; you probably wouldn't eat everything, but simply choose what you want'. The subconscious can be said to be like this: 'it takes what it needs and leaves the rest'. When the time comes for the hypnosis to start, a typical trance induction which I use is as follows:

I would invite you to either sit or lie down and when comfortable to start breathing gently as low down in your stomach as possible, as this always allows the chest to relax, in which there is often a lot of tension. While you are doing this, I'm telling you that whatever you are experiencing is always 100% correct, and you can simply drift off in the way you know that you can, going deeper and deeper into a natural state of relaxation, just enjoying the experience and noticing the relaxation on the outward breath. Very often by now, you are closing your eyes, if not then I suggest that it is easier and easier for your eyes to gradually close. As you are doing this, I begin to talk about the subconscious being the best co-worker that you have within yourself and how it's there to serve you in the very best of ways, giving examples of everyday experiences of how it works for you automatically. I speak with a reassuring tone and rhythm as this promotes both relaxation and reassurance. After 2–3 minutes, I often suggest you can see the number 20 in front of you, and when you can, to gently nod (if you can't, it doesn't matter), then number 19 is slightly smaller and you're going deeper and 18, a little deeper still, and so on taking the numbers backwards — this is what we call 'a deepener'. It only needs a few numbers to allow you to really start to relax. This is often followed on by suggesting 'you close a pair of eyes behind your eyes, and then find a space behind your inner eyes — a place to relax and become aware of the moment of now; the most important moment of all, the past is finished and the future hasn't arrived yet'.

This place you find yourself in is often extremely relaxing, and you are highly 'suggestible' (i.e. positive thoughts, ideas can enter your subconscious from this point onwards very easily). Also 'in the moment of now' ... 'it's the moment that many changes can take place'. This gives you a sense of moving forward and finding whatever you need within yourself to improve the situation you find yourself in. Also for whatever reason, the place behind the inner eyes appears to take the patient to a calmer place within themselves, behind the chaotic thoughts and worries 'in front of their inner eyes'.

So this is a special creative place for a patient to work on themselves, and whatever has been discussed before the trance work can be incorporated at this point. One of the most important points in working with a cancer patient is for them to feel that they have skills to work with.

Hypnotherapeutic Skills

Depending on whether a cancer patient enters therapy, either pre-op or post-op will determine the course of action that I will take with them. When a cancer patient enters therapy before an operation, the course of action is normally to prepare them for the operation itself and help them to deal with the fears surrounding this. One might call this an A and E therapeutic situation, i.e. there is usually very little time to allow the patient to become accustomed to the idea of the operation and help them release the fears around this coming event. There is often what we call 'anticipatory dread' of the operation and fear of the worst outcomes. Very often at a similar time, chemotherapy and/or radiotherapy is given and I find that patients have many contradictory ideas and fears around these clinical interventions. When a patient takes on hypnotherapy in a pre-op situation, I will be looking at ways at reducing these anticipatory fears that the patient has. I will teach them self-hypnosis to help bring a level of calmness and reassurance and there may be skills which can be practiced while the patient is within the self-hypnosis. We may be looking at visualising a successful operation, including feeling and being calm in preparing for it and also a successful outcome. In the hypnotherapy session itself, there would be many reassuring and confidence inspiring suggestions made within the trance work. When the patient repeats the self-hypnosis, some of the feelings and memories of these suggestions can be re-enacted or re-felt, and this helps to continue to boost their confidence and reassurance about the forthcoming operation.

As you would expect, there are so many fears and misconceptions around chemotherapy. Nearly everyone is fearful of it, and many patients think of it as purely poison being introduced into their body. In order to contradict the negativity around these assumptions, it is important for me to look at it in a positive light and express this to my patients. One way I deal with this situation is as follows:

I suggest that the chemotherapy drug is rather like a helper (i.e., it has a specific job to do, and that is to purely focus on the destruction of the cancer). Also, the subconscious works with the chemo to bring about the best affects; in other words, 'they are collaborating' to bring about the best possible results for the patient. While in trance, I often suggest that the patient sees the chemo entering the body in the form of white light, which then targets the exact place of the cancer, while their subconscious directs the appropriate responses within the body. When patients do the self-hypnosis with these visualisations both before and during the chemotherapy, the effects of nausea and negative thinking often is greatly reduced.

Sometimes the anticipatory dread of chemotherapy can be so severe that patients vomit even before entering the hospital. I have found that hypnotherapy is often very powerful in reducing the side effects of chemotherapy before, during and after the administering of the drugs.

I looked after a woman in her forties who came to see me who was very frightened of taking on chemotherapy. Even the thought of going to the hospital made her feel nauseous and she had an ingrained belief that the medication was poison that would be highly detrimental to every part of her body. She was suffering from stage 2 breast cancer, and so it was very necessary for her to take on the treatment. I explained to her that the chemotherapy and her subconscious mind could work together in this treatment, so that the medication would aim completely directly where it was needed, and leave the rest of her body to the care of her subconscious mind. I explained this before we did any trance work. Added to this, I mentioned that while in trance, she would imagine the medication entering her body as white light, which would then go directly to the area which needed the attention. All the rest of her body would be unaffected by this experience. As the lady in question had a spiritual way of thinking, she warmed to these ideas I had mentioned to her and so we started the trance work and incorporated these visualisations. Added to this, she would see herself arriving at the hospital looking calm and confident, then imagine herself doing the self-hypnosis while she was receiving the treatment, and afterwards, imagine she continued to look perfectly okay and ready to go home. We repeated these visualisations several times while she was in hypnosis and she began to feel better and more confident generally. I taught this lady self-hypnosis, so she could practice these tailored visualisations on her own at home before going for her first chemotherapy session. When the day came, she told me she didn't feel nauseous on the way to the hospital, didn't feel ill while receiving the treatment and managed to do self-hypnosis while there. The medication flowed through her body in white light and went straight to the specified location. She felt calm and fell asleep quite quickly. Her attitude to the medication had changed and she believes the side effects had been markedly reduced due to the change in her thought patterns. As she became more confident, it was important for her to continue to practice the self-hypnosis, not only for reducing the side effects of the chemotherapy, but for other aspects as well; for example, to visualise becoming healthier over the coming days and to see herself looking confident, happy and healthy in a few months' time. The main underlying message within the self-hypnosis was that she had the ability to find the resources in herself to improve the way she was feeling and thinking, and that she had some power to improve her circumstances. This acted as an antidote to her feelings of hopelessness and helplessness.

When a patient enters hypnotherapy in a post-operative situation, they are often receiving chemotherapy and sometimes radiotherapy combined. Their emotional and mental state is often quite different than if they had started in a pre-operative situation. They are often in a state of post-operative stress. The body has to overcome the trauma of the operation and their emotions are sometimes in a confused state. On other occasions, the mind may be quite blank and in denial. In either situation, the patient needs to be related to in a very gentle and reassuring way. With a confused or emotional patient, plenty of space and opportunity is required to allow them to express their feelings and help them to make sense of them. Helping them to re-orientate into their surrounding life situation is also important. Cancer is always a life-changing scenario. Many patients say that nothing is ever quite the same after the event. In the case of the traumatised patient, it is very important for me to tread carefully in order that the patient can gradually take on their feelings and memories, so that they can be assimilated in the best possible way.

A woman came to see me who had just been operated on for the removal of one of her ovaries. She was obviously quite stunned by this experience and she needed a lot of support to help her deal with this situation. She was very vague and distant in her communication with me. She had started chemotherapy as well, and one of the difficulties I find is to try and distinguish the symptoms caused by chemotherapy, some of which can be lethargy, aches and pains, nausea, listlessness and depression, as against the patient's emotional reactions to the total cancer experience itself. In this particular case, we worked with the chemotherapy in the way that I mentioned beforehand, and in doing so, we could distinguish the difference between the chemotherapy side effects and that of her emotional response to having had the operation. Helping this patient to reintegrate into her body was the way forward. We allowed her the time to accept and adapt to the changes in her body, and to gradually take on her feelings about her situation in general.

One of the most enjoyable aspects of hypnotherapy is its potential for creative ideas both for the therapist and the patient. Working with cancer patients allows this creative element to come through clearly. Hypnohealing is a good example of this. This is where the belief system of the patient is very important. If the patient has a deeply spiritual belief, then the introduction of the help of masters or guides within the trance work will be especially important to them. This may be associated with a religious interest, for example in Christianity or Buddhism. On a broader perspective, there may be the idea of the power of white light cleansing or clearing the body of cancer. Other patients like the idea of connecting to 'cosmic consciousness', i.e., the energies incoming from the universe. These may be seen as various energies or vibrations. For the more down to earth mind, these ideas may seem outlandish; however, the power of the belief system of a patient shouldn't be underestimated, and is a powerful tool within therapy and a reassuring aspect of it too. Other patients believe that the self-healing comes from within themselves and they can change the way they feel from the internal resources that they have. While in trance, these people may see images of how to deal with their cancer diagnosis. This may be with regards to changes in their diet, directions to work through particular emotional upsets, and finding ways in living a healthier lifestyle in general. I often use hypno-healing when a patient is undergoing chemotherapy. As has already been mentioned, the patient sees the drug going directly to the area affected and gradually destroying the cancer cells, while the rest of the body is completely unaffected by the introduction of the chemotherapy drug.

Hypno-healing and hypno-analysis are very interlinked in the way they often work together. With hypno-analysis, the patient is invited to go into trance and the hypnotherapist asks questions to the patient. I find this is a particularly useful way of working when a patient wants to look at changing their life patterns and how the old ways of living may have contributed to their cancer diagnosis. The calm state of the patient allows their intuition and self-knowledge to come through more easily from their subconscious. In other words, the innate wisdom of the patient has the opportunity to come through while undergoing hypno-analysis. Any number or forms of questions can be asked, and the answers received may be in the form of direct suggestions, pictures or even puzzles that can be unravelled and lead to a successful conclusion.

An example of hypno-analysis might be like this:

'What foods would be beneficial to your body to enhance your immune system?'
'What foods do you need to leave out of your diet?'
'Are there any emotions or unresolved situations which may need to be looked at which could be detrimental to your health?'
The questions sometimes need to be more obscure, for example: 'Go inside and see if you can see the cancer, and do what you need to do to destroy it'.

In a rare number of cases, a patient might want to 'communicate' with the cancer, to find out the message of why it needs to be there at all. As you can imagine, there are any number of questions that can be asked to help the patient find the resources that they need to deal with their situation. Basically in hypno-analysis, it is the body speaking back to both the therapist and the patient from the depths of the subconscious, and how this can be a very powerful healing tool within the therapeutic process. Some patients really enjoy the concept of hypno-analysis. Many women have a deep intuitive knowledge of their mind and body and so the concept and use of hypno-analysis makes a lot of sense to them. It also helps to furnish the idea that the cancer patient has a lot more control over the way think and can have a better understanding about what is going on within them.

A couple of years ago, a woman came to see me who had been diagnosed with stage 1 breast cancer and in general she was very fearful. Although it had been explained that her life was not in danger, she couldn't quite believe this, and so part of the job in the therapy was to try and reassure her that her future was very positive and she had so many things to look forward to. She was happily married and she had a very supportive husband. She had a creative background and so found hypnosis both interesting and in many ways enjoyable. While undergoing hypno-analysis, she realised that she needed a powerful guide in her whom she could trust and rely on. His job would be to oversee the healthiness of her immune system, and he would be in 'a control room' somewhere deep within her. He would oversee her health at night and help her to sleep. As the weeks progressed, her confidence increased and she felt she had found both guidance and support within herself. As can be seen, hypno-analysis has the ability to give direction and strength in any number of ways to the person who needs extra support or a deeper understanding of themselves.

One of the most difficult scenarios that many women have to go through is their fear of pain, whether it be after the operation, or as a result of radiotherapy, and of course in terminal cases, the level of pain that may have to be faced before death. Sometimes there is no pain at all before diagnosis and it's a great shock to have been given a cancer diagnosis. In all these cases, the fact that pain is felt enhances the negative experience as many of you will already know; especially as pain continually highlights the discomfort, both physically and emotionally, which you may be going through.

Hypnotherapy can look at pain from both an emotional and physical point of view. The experience of pain often results in women feeling separate and detached from the area in which they are suffering. I have found that women who have been suffering from cancers in the pelvic area often feel completely separated from the area in question. I remember asking one woman who was being treated for ovarian cancer whether she felt connected to her pelvic area. She replied, 'I feel as if my genitals are on the other side of the room'. As you can imagine, this reply somewhat shocked me; however, I could see in one respect that this was a coping strategy, but it was important for her to reconnect to this area at some point, in order that self-healing could be more powerfully introduced; also, to help her let go of the trauma experienced. It was important also to reconnect to her genital area to bring back the ability for her to have sexual relations with her partner. Sometimes the intensity of pain is greatly increased due to the emotional component of it. In the above case, she felt generalised pain in the pelvic area, a long time after the removal of her ovary.

In working with reconnecting her closeness and awareness of her pelvic region, she felt much calmer and the pain was greatly reduced, with the result that she resumed sexual relations with her partner.

Separation from the area of the body, which is suffering, is quite a natural response and is a way of helping a person deal with their discomfort. I have outlined below a few techniques that I use to help to alleviate pain and which some of you might be interested in practicing yourselves. One of the decisions that I have to make is to decide whether to use a 'dissociation technique', i.e., to separate the patient further from the pain, which can be useful with 'intractable pain' when the person is in distress and has to escape from it. This method of separating the patient from the pain is sometimes used when medication doesn't appear to modify it. Another way to deal with pain is to change the nature of it. If you can think now of a pain that you may be suffering from, and imagine the 'feeling' quality of it changing, how much better might that feel for you. Imagine changing a raw burning sensation to a softer flowing warm feeling. This can be achieved through hypnotic work and as you can imagine is a very useful way of relieving the emotional and physical discomfort within pelvic pain. In order to achieve this, it is necessary for the patient to be connected to the area suffering from pain. Another method I use is to help the person understand what the pain is trying to tell them (i.e., work with it and see if a change in lifestyle, habits or maybe diet can affect the intensity of it). Also, a negative previous experience may need to be released in order for the pain to be reduced.

When I work with the relationship the patient has with their pain, then the experience of the pain itself can change. Once again, when the idea of the subconscious is considered as a co-worker, then the patient can feel less overwhelmed by the discomfort and can find various resources from within themselves to help them deal with it.

When a person is in hypnosis, I often introduce the idea of a pain scale where the higher the number the worse the pain is being felt and so in asking the patient to lower the number accessed, this is giving a clear message to lower the intensity of the discomfort. As you can imagine, this helps the patient feel more in control of their pain and to enhance the view concerning the value of their subconscious and how this changes the way they are experiencing their pain.

As I am sure you all realise, there are so many external factors that you have to deal with in being a cancer patient. How to approach the subject with your family and friends is often a big issue. The timing of this is important as well. Finding the right moment to broach the subject and how to go about it often causes a considerable amount of distress. Naturally, others' reactions to a cancer diagnosis will sometimes be surprising as well. Some people will stay away, while others may well be emotional and even inappropriate in their responses. So all types of reactions need to be taken into account, thus psychological and practical support can be supplied by the hypnotherapist. Both within and out of hypnosis a 'mental rehearsal' of how to deal with these reactions is often useful, and also to help the patient take the time they need to deal with their own feelings and experiences

One of the most surprising conversations that sometimes comes up is how their cancer has changed their life in a positive way, i.e., to look at their life from a new perspective and to consider the more important aspects of it. One lady who had been diagnosed with stage 1 cancer of the breast decided she would take life less seriously and really enjoy her free time instead of continuously working virtually 24 hours a day. She felt that years of deep stress and anxiety might have been a contributory cause for her diagnosis. Now, she thoroughly enjoys self-hypnosis, and is highly creative in her approach to the exercises which she has created within it. She has been free of cancer for several years now and is enjoying life so much more.

Other women I have come across sometimes look back over their lives and wonder where they went wrong and have feelings of guilt concerning 'bringing on' their cancer diagnosis. In other words, they feel they have brought this on themselves. This a very tricky area and needs to be dealt with great sensitivity. The last thing a person needs to feel is guilty for having cancer! It is very important not to jump to conclusions too. In other words, to suggest that a major trauma experienced sometime before diagnosis is the reason for the onset of the cancer. Another example would be that unresolved anger over a number of years was definitely the catalyst that set the cancer in motion. In one case that I have come across, a woman who had stage 2 endometrial cancer felt that this had been brought on by years of anger and frustration due to an earlier history of sexual abuse in her childhood. This had resulted in pent-up anger and rage trapped in her pelvic area, which could not be appropriately expressed, and hence these internalised negative emotions had manifested into cancer. She felt she hadn't taken the opportunity to undertake therapy to release these emotions at a much earlier time in her life, and had she done so, this cancer diagnosis would never have manifested. It wouldn't have been appropriate for me to contradict this assumption, but rather instead to work with it, because it was in her belief system, and it wasn't for me to make a judgment either way.

Basically, if patients believe that negative experiences in their past have contributed to their cancer diagnosis; to help them overcome their emotional distress is a useful way of working with the patient as part of the therapeutic plan. Also, a patient's intuition or innate wisdom often serves them well, and should never be discounted by any therapist.

One of the most challenging and difficult situations to work with is the terminal cancer case, especially if an inoperable situation arises while in the middle of therapy. I used to make a home visit to a lady who was suffering from multiple cancers. It started with ovarian cancer and then she developed endometrial cancer as well. This required a complete hysterectomy. Unfortunately, in the following months, the cancer spread through her organs, including her pancreas, and by that time her situation was inoperable and she had to come to terms with the outlook of only being given a few months to live. At the start of the therapy she felt that despite all odds, she could beat the cancer and eventually become well again. We worked with reducing the side effects of the chemotherapy as well as other stress reducing techniques. She had the opportunity to really discuss in detail her life and where she felt she might have gone wrong. She felt there wasn't much depth to her life and that she had completed what she had come into life to do. There were severe family confrontations which had not been dealt with, but she felt she couldn't do anything about this. Although her husband was very supportive, she knew he wanted to take a totally different direction in life, which to some extent would be at odds with hers. As time passed, she began to accept the finality of her situation. The subject of how to deal with her impending death had to be broached at some point, and the timing of this was of ultimate importance. On a particular day, we both knew that the subject needed to be spoken about honestly and openly. It was as if there was a sudden change in the atmosphere of the session. A calmness came over her as we spoke about it. She felt she didn't need to struggle any more. She wanted to just rest and gradually let go. This lady was not religious in any way, and didn't have any definite thoughts about an afterlife. She just wanted to settle her affairs and drift away into a sense of peace. This is where hypnosis can be very useful.

There can almost be a multi-dimensional feel about it. Within self-hypnosis creative visualisations can bring about a sense of peace, and being able to escape from the chaos and worries of the world. In the last few sessions, she learnt techniques within hypnosis of detaching her mind from her body so she could escape the discomfort she was suffering from and go to a spiritual place that was beyond her body into a world of peacefulness and beauty. She felt she was not alone in making these journeys, and this seemed to awaken a spiritual awareness in her. By this time, I was a kind of guide to help her reach these 'special places' in her mind. A gradual quietness and acceptance of her situation came to her and when the time came, I believe she left this world in as a peaceful way as possible. As a therapist and a human being, I feel it is a great honour and learning experience to help a person leave this physical world and move on to another level of existence. There can be a level of deep sharing which personally I feel is barely matched in any other situation in life, and I find it challenges my own belief system and helps me to have a broader understanding of the value of life in general.

I am sure that many of you readers would agree that one of the most difficult situations that a woman has to deal with is a sense of losing part of her femininity after having had either a mastectomy or hysterectomy, and hypnotherapy is one course of action that can be taken in order to help alleviate these feelings of loss. The most obvious situation where this arises is when a woman has just had a total hysterectomy and she knows it is impossible from that point on to bear children. This is especially diffi-cult when she feels that having a family was the goal she most desired in life. This feeling of a loss of femininity is often associated with those feel-ings I mentioned earlier on concerning being detached from the pelvic area. I have often found that a physical detachment from the area operated on, and feelings of a loss of femininity often go hand in hand. Because of this, I find it's very important to be extra careful and sensitive in my approach in working with these patients. Sometimes, a woman may feel a sense of 'deadness' in both their mind and body, as this amnesia-type response is a way for them to deal with their circumstances. However, there comes a time when emotional and physical integration needs to take place in order that the patient has the possibility to move on in their life. A lady came to see me with ovarian cancer and had one ovary removed six months previously, the result of which she felt both separated from her pelvic area and had also lost part of her femininity. She said her pelvic area felt numb and lifeless and she had not been able to resume a sexual rela-tionship with her partner as her libido had fallen to zero. She said there was a sense of loss and she was worried about the future, as well as the feelings of her partner who had been very supportive. She discussed her situation in great detail and I realised that she had a 'spiritual dimension' in her belief system. She believed in the power of prayer, the value of meditation and how visualisations could help her. This open-mindedness allowed me to access a wide range of therapeutic tools to work with. She enjoyed hypnosis and found it very relaxing, and she could access her sub-conscious easily. This allowed her to go into her own intuitive feelings about how to move forward and this gave me clues in the direction to fol-low within the therapeutic work. Naturally she was worried about recon-necting to her pelvic area, as she felt that the emotional pain and loss would be too much to bear. However, in strengthening her own self-healing abilities within hypnosis and self-hypnosis, she could 'invite' her pelvic area back into her body and it would be 'embraced and accepted' by the whole of her body and psyche as well. In addition to this, we looked at how 'other aspects of her femininity' could be looked at and strengthened and would come to her help in re-establishing a feminine harmonisation in herself. The idea of a rising phoenix can be very powerful in this work. The result of this work brought feelings of integration, a resumed life-force in her pelvic area and a gradual increase in her sex libido. As the months progressed, she felt her femininity had begun to increase, and sexual relations with her partner had resumed. It can be seen from this that the loss felt by this woman was so much more than the removal of her ovary, but extended well beyond this into other areas of her life as well.

Returning to Normality

After a period of time when all the regular check-ups are clear and the initial shock and trauma of the cancer diagnosis is well past, there comes a time when the idea of 'returning to normality' can be brought into the therapy sessions. Many patients go through long periods of intense feelings about their cancer situation, and naturally this often overtakes their life in many respects. What is important here is to get the right timing. If it is necessary to continue to offload deep emotional worries and fears, then it would be inappropriate for me to talk about returning to normality at this point. This is because my patient may well view this as their emotional turmoil being trivialised by me. However, when the time is right, and this is often an intuitive feeling felt both by the therapist and patient, then the idea of returning to a normal life can be a very beneficial way of working. This can boost confidence for the patient, and help them put 'cancer into the past', so they can move on from being 'an ill patient' to 'a well patient'. There is so much at stake in this transition. When a woman feels she is truly well, it is incredibly reassuring for her. It means that all the time that they 'were worrying', can now be put into a more positive use. There comes with it a sense of freedom and at last control back in their life. It means they no longer need to feel they are a victim of their cancer and many of the labels associated with having cancer can be let go of, e.g., 'I'm a victim', 'I can never be well again'. This letting go of labels gives a person so much more space to take on various ideas, projects and maybe have the impetus to take on something new, which beforehand they would not have had the courage or dynamism to do. When I am working with someone at this stage, there are lots of suggestions of 'forward thinking' within the hypnosis and the idea of cancer is deeply relegated to the past, almost as if it was in a different life, and there can be a time when it feels like this. I often suggest that they continue with self-hypnosis as this is beneficial to their health in general.

One of the main objectives of this chapter has been to show you some of the techniques available within hypnotherapy in how to manage cancer. More importantly, however, is that your own self-healing capabilities can be realised through the use of self-hypnosis. In other words, there is an 'internal healer' within yourself, which has the ability to surface and help you on your journey to recovery.

There is such an array of hypnotherapy organisations out there; however, all hypnotherapists registered with the General Hypnotherapy Register have a sound training. Also, the General Hypnotherapy Standards Council has a list of organisations which would be of help to you. The Society of Medical and Dental Hypnotherapists also has a comprehensive list of hypnotherapists available to you.

Chapter 16

Nutrition by Nigel Denby

If you search the internet for diet and cancer, you'll get over 140 million snippets of information at your fingertips in a matter of seconds. Some will be useful, some won't. Some will be based on sound science, some on anecdote and some on complete pseudo-science. Some may even be downright dangerous and could lead to serious nutritional deficiency or interfere with cancer treatment.

So, to save you having to wade through the mass and from trying to sort the wheat from the chaff, the next few pages will take you through the latest evidence based dietary advice for preventing cancer and improving the outcome if you already have cancer.

It's an undeniable fact that what you eat and how much you weigh most definitely has an impact on your risk of getting cancer. Diet also has a huge impact on your outcome if you are one of the 1 in 3 of us who develops some form of the disease.

You really are what you eat; an incredible 40% of cancers could be prevented by diet and lifestyle — so what have you got to lose by giving eating well a try?

The World Cancer Research Fund suggests a list of recommendations about diet and for me these are good starting point:

- Be as lean as possible without becoming underweight.
- Be physically active for at least 30 minutes every day.
- Avoid sugar drinks and limit your intake of energy or calorie-dense foods.

- Eat more vegetables, fruits, whole grains and legumes such as beans and lentils.
- Limit your intake of red meat like beef, pork and lamb and avoid processed meats.
- Limit your alcohol intake to 2 units per day for men and 1 unit per day for women.
- Limit your consumption of salty foods.
- Don't take supplements to protect against cancer.

That all might sound very familiar, but putting it all into practice can be a tall order so let's look a little closer at each step and get practical about the anti-cancer diet.

Be as Lean as Possible

Being a healthy weight is second only to not smoking as the most important thing that can be done for cancer prevention.

World Cancer research Fund.

Are you a healthy weight for your height? About 1 in 5 adults in the UK today are heavy enough to increase their risk of cancer. There are several ways of checking whether your current weight or body shape is likely to affect your health. These include working out your body mass index (BMI) and checking your waist size. Please note the measurements given here are for adults over 18 years.

Measuring your BMI is a useful way of finding out whether your weight is putting your health at risk. Your BMI, a measure that is used by health professionals around the world, is based on your height and weight and can be worked out by dividing your weight (in kilograms) by your height (in metres) squared. You can find a complete reference table at NHS Livewell: http://www.nhs.uk/Livewell/healthy-living/Pages/height-weight-chart.aspx.

For any height, there is a range of healthy weights. BMI is classified in the following way:

- **Less than 18.5 kg/m^2** You are underweight. You may need to gain weight.

- **18.5 to 24.9 kg/m^2** You are a healthy weight and should aim to stay that way.
- **25 to 29.9 kg/m^2** This level of BMI is defined as overweight. It's a good idea to lose some weight for your health's sake, or at least aim to prevent further weight gain. A good target for weight loss for you will be between 6.5 kg–13 kg (1–2 stone) over 3–4 months. Even a weight loss of just 3% of your starting weight will help to reduce your health risk.
- **Over 30 kg/m^2** This level is defined as obese and your health is at risk. Losing weight will improve your health. A good initial target for weight loss would be 13 kg (2 stone), although you may need to lose a little more than this to achieve a healthy BMI.
- **Over 40 kg/m^2** You may need specialist help to manage your weight and health. This is especially important before taking up any new exercise.

Note: BMI is not always a good reflection of body fatness. A very muscular person might have a high BMI when in fact their body fat is at a healthy level, as muscle weighs more than fat.

Waist measurements and what they mean

It would also be a good idea to take some measurements like waist, hips and bust or chest. To take measurements use a flexible tape measure and make sure you measure the same spot each time. Keep the tape measure straight for the most accurate results.

- Waist — measure around the naval or belly button
- Hips — measure at the widest point of your bottom
- Bust or chest — measure around the widest point

Waist measurement is a good indicator of your fat distribution, which is linked to cancer risk. Carrying too much weight around your middle is a sign that you're at increased risk of developing some cancers, as well as heart disease, high blood pressure and diabetes.

People who carry excess weight around their middle are often referred to as 'apple shaped', whereas those who carry the weight on their hips are 'pear shaped'. Women are usually pear shaped, while men are more likely to be apple shaped. Measuring your waist is an easy way of finding out

	At increased risk	At high risk
European men	94 cm (37 in) Aim to lose between 1 and 2 stones or 6.5 kg to 13 kg.	102 cm (40 in) Aim to lose at least 2 stones or 13 kg
Asian men	90 cm (36 in) Aim to lose between 1 and 2 stones or 6.5 kg to 13 kg	96 cm (38 in) Aim to lose at least 2 stones or 13 kg
All women	80 cm (32 in) Aim to lose between 1 and 2 stones or 6.5 kg to 13kg	88 cm (35 in) Aim to lose at least 2 stones or 13 kg

Figure 16.1   Waist measurement.

whether you're an 'apple' or a 'pear'. Use the table below to see if you are at risk of ill health. Remember, these measurements refer to adults, not children.

If you are at increased risk, now would be a good time to make healthy lifestyle changes that would reduce or prevent any further increase. If you are at high risk, then losing weight and reducing your waist size would improve your health.

If you are working to increase your day-to-day activity levels, then measurements will be especially important to you, because you may well change shape and lose inches faster than you lose weight. This is because as you increase your activity level, you replace some fat with muscle and muscle is heavier than fat. This increase in muscle tissue is exactly what you want. More muscle tissue results in a faster metabolic rate and that means you burn more calories even when you're asleep. And, you guessed it, burning more calories means that you lose weight more easily!

A general guide for a healthy weekly weight loss is between ¼ kg and 1 kg ($\frac{1}{2}$ lb to 2 lb a week) or anything up to 1 kg per week.

Be Physically Active for at least 30 Minutes Every Day

Being active is a really important part of your anti-cancer diet and will help you stay in control of your weight and your health for a lifetime. Remember an old-fashioned set of grocer's scales — Now imagine putting the things you eat on one side of the scales and the things you do to burn energy on the other side. How balanced is your lifestyle?

More energy in than going out = Weight gain

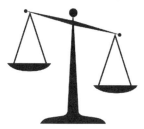

Equal amounts of energy in and energy out = weight maintenance

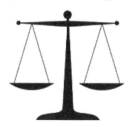

More energy out than going in = weight loss

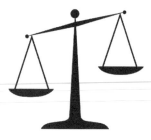

Of course, there are several ways to shift the balance in favour of weight loss:

- You can put all your energy into exercising, so you can get away with eating anything you like without gaining weight. (I could never love exercise this much, so I'd say no thanks!)
- You can restrict your eating to such an extent that you make all the calorie savings you need to lose weight without lifting a finger. (I love eating too much to do that.)

- **Or you can take an altogether more reasonable approach and choose to save a few calories here and burn a few off there. (Now that sounds more like it!)**

Don't panic: you don't have to race out and sign up to the gym. But you do need to take regular physical activity (it can just be daily walking!) as part of your anti-cancer diet. Making simple changes to fit activity into your everyday routine does take a bit of getting used to, I admit. But after a couple of weeks it will feel like the norm, believe me — and you'll wonder why you found it so hard before.

Being active can become so normal to you that it won't take long before you'll miss it if you don't do something every day. I've said you never have to set foot in a gym to keep fit. But of course, if you enjoy a workout don't let me stop you. Just make sure your gym sessions are a bonus on top of your daily activity routine.

Here's a challenge for you so you can see for yourself. Start taking a brisk 30-minute walk, or some other activity, every day for two weeks. I'll guarantee that it will help feel much more like you really want to and feel. Will you take the challenge?

And here's the best bit. You can choose to break up the 30 minutes if you want you could do 10:10:10 minutes, 5:20:5 minutes or 15:15 minutes. That is, you can take your exercise all in one go, or in three segments of different time lengths throughout the day — it's entirely up to you. Two lots of 15 minutes of brisk walking will do you just as much good as one lot of 30 minutes. It's the fact that you're doing it and, most importantly, doing it every day that matters.

Just 30 minutes' brisk activity every day will do a lot to move you towards your health goals. It will encourage your body to make new lean, muscle tissue, which means your metabolic rate will speed up and you'll burn more calories even when you're asleep.

Avoid Sugar Drinks and Limit your Intake of Energy or Calorie-Dense Foods

Sugar gives the body energy and, of course, helps make sweet foods taste good. The sugars in our diet come from lots of different sources: some of them are obvious, like the refined white sugar you sprinkle on cornflakes or stir into a cup of tea; others are less obvious and can be lurking where you might not expect to find them. For example, there are naturally occurring sugars in things like fruit, fruit juice and milk, or foods that we don't necessarily think of as being sweet, like baked beans, tomato ketchup or bread and pasta. While most of us like the taste of having *some* sugar in our diet, it's important not to overdo it — but most of us do! Too much sugar is bad news for your teeth and your waistline. The sugar that occurs naturally in foods like fruit and milk is less of a problem, because it arrives with a whole host of other nutritional goodies, such as antioxidant vitamins (A, C, E and beta carotene) and calcium. The sugar to be wary of is the white stuff and the hidden sugars. Nutritionists and dieticians tend to class added sugar as 'empty calories' — that's calories which don't provide any other real nutritional benefits. Empty calories = added body fat.

Most adults in the UK eat too much sugar, so we should all be trying to eat fewer sugary foods, such as sweets, cakes and biscuits, and to drink fewer soft drinks.

Sugar is added to many types of food, such as:

- fizzy drinks and juice drinks
- sweets and biscuits
- jam
- cakes, pastries and puddings
- ice cream

What about fruit juice?

The sugars found naturally in whole fruit are less likely to cause tooth decay than are refined sugars because they are contained within the structure of the fruit. But when fruit is juiced or blended, the sugars are released. Once released, these sugars can damage teeth, much like other sugars, especially if fruit juice is drunk frequently.

Fruit juice is a healthy choice and counts towards the five portions of fruit and vegetables we should be having every day, but it is best to drink fruit juice at mealtimes and stick to one small glass per day.

Tips for cutting down on your sugar intake

If you have a sweet tooth and are trying to reduce your sugar intake, these tips might help you cut down:

- Have fewer sugary drinks and snacks.
- Instead of sugary fizzy drinks and juice drinks, choose water or unsweetened fruit juice.
- If you like fizzy drinks, then try diluting fruit juice with sparkling water.
- Instead of cakes or biscuits, try having a currant bun, scone or some malt loaf with low-fat spread.
- If you take sugar in hot drinks, or add sugar to your breakfast cereal, gradually reduce the amount until you can cut it out altogether. Eventually, your taste buds won't miss it.
- Rather than spreading jam, marmalade, syrup, treacle or honey on your toast, try a low-fat spread, sliced banana or low-fat cream cheese instead.
- Use food labels to help you CHECK, COMPARE and CHOOSE the foods with less added sugar.
- Try halving the sugar you use in your own recipes. It works for most things.
- Choose tins of fruit in juice rather than syrup.
- Choose wholegrain breakfast cereals or porridge rather than those coated with sugar or honey, or try a mix of half and half.

Eat more vegetables, fruits, whole grains and legumes such as beans and lentils and limit your intake of red meat like beef, pork and lamb and avoid processed meats.

Plant Foods and Cancer Prevention

Basing your diet on plant foods (like whole grains, pulses such as beans, vegetables and fruits), which contain fibre and other nutrients, can reduce our cancer risk. These foods contain plenty of fibre and water and tend to be lower in energy-density which means they can help us to maintain a healthy weight. Now, this doesn't mean you need to become a vegetarian; it just means you shift the emphasis from animal foods to plant foods — it's a very simple, but amazingly affective diet shift which brings some extraordinary health benefits.

Research shows that vegetables and fruits probably protect against a range of cancers, including:

- mouth, pharynx and larynx
- oesophagus
- stomach
- lung

Recent research into bowel cancer found strong evidence that foods containing dietary fibre decrease the risk of bowel cancer. These foods include wholegrain bread and pasta, and oats. Fibre is thought to have many benefits, including helping to speed up how quickly food moves through our digestive system.

Vegetables and fruits may protect against cancer because they contain vitamins and minerals, which help keep your body healthy and strengthen your immune system. They are also sources of phytochemicals like anti-oxidants. These can help to protect cells in your body from damage that can lead to cancer. Plant foods can also help you to maintain a healthy weight because most of them help keep you feeling full, but are low in energy or calorie density compared to other foods like meat and dairy foods.

What are plant foods?

Broadly speaking, plant foods fit into these main categories. Aim to eat these types of foods with every meal. Try to fill two-thirds of your plate with plant foods and just one-third with animal foods (see Figure 16.2) — it's that simple!

Wholegrain foods and pulses

- whole grains (cereals) — including rice, oats, pasta and bread
- pulses — such as lentils, chickpeas and beans

Vegetables and fruits

Starchy foods such as:
- roots and tubers — including potatoes and yams

PLANT BASED EATING

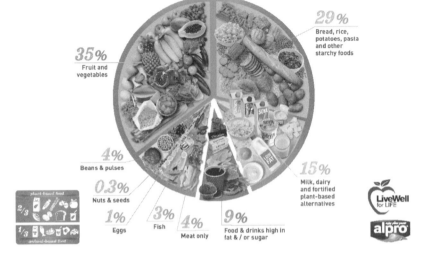

Figure 16.2 Plant-based eating.

Non-wholegrain foods

- white rice, pasta and bread

  Remember, base your anti-cancer diet around whole grains, pulses, vegetable and fruits.

What is a 5 A DAY portion?

Almost all vegetables and fruits count, apart from starchy tubers and roots like potatoes, yam, sweet potatoes and cassava. You can even use frozen, dried and canned vegetables and fruits. The more variety the better.

As a rough guide, a portion is:

- Three heaped tablespoons of cooked vegetables like broccoli or carrots.
- A small cereal bowl of salad vegetables like lettuce or spinach.
- A medium-sized piece of fruit like an apple or a banana.
- A slice of large fruit like melon.
- A handful of smaller fruit like grapes.

Table 16.1   Plant based Vs animal based meals and snacks.

Higher calorie density foods	Lower calorie density plant based foods	By swapping to the plant based lower calorie density option….
2 × chocolate hobnobs 38 g	Large handful of cherries 100 g	↑More than double the volume of food ↓70% fewer calories (184 Kcals vs. 55 Kcals)
Cheese (30 g) and 2 cream crackers with butter	50g low fat hummus with crudités	↑ 6 times the volume of food (56 g vs. 325 g) 37% fewer calories (262 Kcals vs. 191K cals)
50 g granola with dollop of Greek yoghurt and 2 tsp honey	50 g muesli with soya fruit yoghurt and 80 g mixed berries	↑11% more volume of food ↓1/3rd fewer calories (409 Kcals vs. 274Kcals)
125 g serving of beef mince	50:50 mix of 75 g lean minced beef with 75 g mushrooms and 50 g green lentils	↑60% more volume of food ↓more than 1/3rd fewer calories (263 Kcals vs. 168 Kcals)

- A tablespoon of dried fruit like raisins.
- Two small fruit like satsumas or plums.
- Three heaped tablespoons of pulses, e.g. chickpeas or baked beans — but pulses only count as one portion a day, no matter how much you eat.
- A small glass (150 ml) of pure fruit juice — but again fruit juice only counts as one portion a day, no matter how much you drink.

If you need more convincing that basing your diet on plant foods is a good move, just look at these simple swaps and how you get to eat more food with more fibre for less calories and fat. Table 16.1 makes some suggestions on what you can swap in your diet.

Animal foods are not the enemy

You really don't need to cut all animal foods out of your diet. Meat, fish, poultry, eggs and dairy foods contain a lot of really good, important nutrients. The fact is though, that most of us eat far more animal foods than we need and not enough plant foods — so this switch in emphasis is about re-balancing your diet. So, still enjoy:

- Scrambled eggs for breakfast — just have them less often and serve them with some grilled tomatoes and mushrooms and whole grain toast instead of bacon and sausages — or try a Quorn™ sausage!
- A nice grilled steak — aim to have no more than about 500 g red meat each week and try to stay away from processed meats as much as possible.
- Roast chicken — poultry is low in fat as long as you don't eat the skin. Have plenty of veggies and potatoes with your Sunday Roast and use the 1/3:2/3 plate model to help you keep the balance right.
- Fish remains a really healthy food — aim for at least two servings a week: one white fish like cod, haddock or sole, and one oily fish like salmon, trout, mackerel or canned sardines.
- You can still enjoy Shepherd's pie or spaghetti bolognaise, but use a little less minced beef or lamb and mix it with some chopped mushrooms and green lentils.
- Try some alternatives to dairy milk, cream, yoghurt and custards.

Alcohol

Limit your alcohol intake to 2 units per day for men and 1 unit per day for women.

Alcohol contains what nutritionists call 'empty calories'. These are calories that have absolutely no nutritional value: no vitamins, minerals, fibre or protein. Alcohol contains 7 calories per gram, which puts it second only to fat, at 9 calories per gram, in high calorific value.

Let's imagine you have two large glasses of wine each evening. That's 330 empty calories each night; or 2,310 empty calories in one week. Most adults only need between 2000 kcals and 2500 kcals per day. That means you would be drinking more than one days' worth of calories per week, in booze alone. If you enjoy the occasional drink, then there is no need to give up alcohol altogether, but if you want to be healthy, you must be aware of the contribution your alcohol intake has on your total calorie intake.

Table 16.2 shows the calorie values and alcohol units for a selection of popular drinks at standard pub measures.

Table 16.2   Calorie values of popular alcoholic drinks.

Alcoholic drink	Calories
Large glass dry white wine (2 units)	165
$\frac{1}{2}$ pint regular strength lager (1 unit)	65
Gin and tonic (1unit)	114
Vodka and orange juice (1 unit)	164
Southern Comfort and lemonade (1 unit)	193
Tia Maria and coke (1 unit)	180
Medium glass of red wine (1$\frac{1}{2}$ units)	119
$\frac{1}{2}$ pint of cider (1 unit)	103
Glass of champagne (1 unit)	95

It's recommended that you have at least two or three alcohol-free days each week. These tips can help you reduce the amount you drink and the calories you consume through alcohol:

- If you drink wine, try changing to wine spritzers, made with half wine and half soda water or sparkling mineral water.
- Use diet mixers with spirits.
- Choose lager or bitter shandy made with diet lemonade instead regular beer.
- Alternate an alcoholic drink with a diet soft drink or sparkling mineral water.
- Offer to drive to the pub so you can't drink!

Salt

Limit your consumption of salty foods.

The white stuff you sprinkle on your chips is known to most of us as table salt, but when it comes to food labels, salt will often be shown using its chemical name: sodium chloride. Sodium is an essential mineral required by the body. One of its functions is to help balance the levels of fluid in the body, which helps to maintain normal blood pressure and keep nerves and muscles working properly. However, an excessive intake of sodium may cause problems for some people and a medical debate links sodium intake with stomach cancer and high blood pressure (hypertension).

Confusing labelling

Most packaged food products carry a nutrition label on the back of the pack that, in line with current legislation, states the sodium content rather than the salt content — which isn't really that helpful. To work out the equivalent amount of salt, multiply the sodium value by 2.5 (e.g. 1.2 g sodium is equivalent to 3.0 g salt). Some packs also provide a 'salt equivalent' figure based on this calculation, as shown in this example.

NUTRITIONAL INFORMATION for chicken and vegetable bake		
Typical values	per 100g	per 350g pack
Energy-kJ	480kJ	1680 kJ
- kcal	115 kcal	405 kcal
Protein	9.5 g	33.3 g
Carbohydrate	8.6 g	30.1 g
of which sugars	3.5 g	12.3 g
Fat	4.6 g	16.1 g
of which saturates	2.0 g	7.0 g
Fibre	1.5 g	5.3 g
Sodium*	0.3 g	1.1 g
*Equivalent as salt	0.8 g	2.8 g

Sodium — what's high or low?

The Food Standards Agency (FSA) recommends the following guidelines:

High   0.6 g sodium or more per 100 g of food
Low   0.1 g sodium or less per 100 g of food

However, take account of the portion size of the food you eat to help gauge the amount of sodium. For example, certain foods, such as yeast extracts, are relatively high in sodium at 45 g per 100 g, but are eaten in very small quantities as an average serving is 4 g, which means you'd actually be eating 1.8 g per serving.

Tips for cutting down on your salt intake

Shopping

- Check the nutrition labels to keep track of your salt and sodium intake.
- Look for 'reduced salt' or 'reduced sodium' advice on packs. These foods should be at least 25% lower in salt than the standard product. Opt for reduced-salt versions of foods whenever possible, including bread, baked beans, crisps, biscuits, butter, fat spreads, soups, gravy granules, crackers and ready meals.
- Choose canned vegetables marked 'no added salt' and products such as tuna that are canned in water rather than brine.
- Try using low-sodium salt substitutes for use in cooking and at the table (but don't use these if you have kidney problems).
- Cut down on inherently salty foods: cured meat, cheese, smoked meat and fish, olives, anchovies and soy sauce.

Cooking

- Aim to reduce the amount of salt used in cooking — do this gradually, as your taste buds may take time to adjust.
- If a recipe tells you to reduce the volume of a stock, add the seasoning after the reducing stage, rather than before.
- Experiment! We all want tasty food, so replace salt with other flavours. Try different herbs such as basil, chives, lemon grass, rosemary or coriander, and spices such as chilli, ginger, garlic or cumin.
- Taste your food before adding salt at the table, and then take just a little if needed.

Eating out

- When your food arrives, taste it before adding salt. If you feel more salt is needed, add only a little.
- Moderate the amount of sauces you add, such as soy sauce, as they can be high in salt.

You don't have to stop eating foods that are higher in salt, as all foods can fit into a healthy balanced diet. However, if you eat several high-salt foods, cut back the salt in other foods at other times to maintain a balance.

Supplements

Don't take supplements to protect against cancer. It's estimated that around 10% of cancer patients take high doses of nutritional supplements — especially antioxidant supplements like Beta Carotene, vitamin C, vitamin E and selenium. It's perfectly understandable to want to do anything and everything to try and improve the outcome of cancer.

When it comes to diet and nutrition, prevention is all about what you do most of the time over a long period of time. There really are no quick fixes. If you want to take one multivitamin and mineral supplement a day as an insurance policy for days when you don't eat quite as well as you'd planned, that's fine. But taking high dose single supplements is not recommended at all. At best, it's a waste of money, and at worst, it could even be harmful to you.

Although some studies have shown that high dose supplements have possibly reduced the nasty side effects of some cancer treatments, there are also a number of good studies which also show these supplements protect cancer cells from the very treatments which are given to kill them.

When it comes to supplements, remember they can never make a bad diet healthy; they can never replace a healthy diet and above all, supplements are not Smarties — they too can have their own side effects.

Chapter 17

Cardiac Synchronicity, the Secular Approach to Chant: How might understanding the heart's role in our emotional responses apply to the 4 cusp approach? by Dr Tony Yardley-Jones

Editorial note from JRS: This chapter has come about because of an interesting juxtaposition of ideas. Shaun Hammond and I were discussing the difference in mental state between hypnotic trance and the place of otherness that one can reach by repetitive chant where the chant is in time with the heart beat and breathing. They feel similar, but are not the same. Tony happened to join the conversation and in great excitement told about a technique called cardiac synchronicity; this is a secular approach to repetitive prayer.

The 'Emotional' Heart in History

Traditionally, Western medicine has regarded the heart primarily as a mechanical pump unrelated to our psychological or emotional life. This is very different to the symbolic depiction of the heart as the primary seat or source of emotion, which has existed across centuries, for example, in literature, music and other forms of art. That 'mechanical' view is, however, changing.

Through the emergence of scientific explanations for the link between mind and body and the heart and emotions, the heart is beginning to recapture the emotional essence of its past.

Neuroscientific findings over the last 20 years have revealed how the neural networks of both heart and brain generate signals that impact and influence each other's functioning. Research has shown how the heart is a crucial part of a complex mind–body system. Intricate, dynamic responses and feedback loops exist between the heart and brain, involving other aspects of the nervous system as well. Research on individual heart data is also found to be a powerful indicator of the health effects resulting from negative and positive emotions.

Research groups have focused on exploring *how* and *why* positive emotions improve health and, specifically, on uncovering physiological correlates of positive emotional states that may help explain these observations. Since so many different emotions occur during the journey anyone undertakes as they move through the cusp approach to a cancer diagnosis, the question arises as to whether the body has mechanisms to deal with and change emotional states? Is it possible to move to a positive emotional state, thereby optimising on the psychological, physiological and 'healing' benefits associated with such positive emotional states? What role does the heart play in such processes and can an individual harness that mechanism?

In this chapter, I have tried to outline how understanding emotion-related changes in the patterns of the heart's rhythmic activity and heart–brain interactions naturally affect physiological, emotional and thinking processes. Furthermore, I will describe how they can be influenced, with training, to capture those benefits at a time when 'feeling positive' may be the most difficult state to attain.

How does the Heart Physiologically Influence Emotional Processes?

It is now recognised that the brain and body work in conjunction in order for perceptions, thoughts, and emotions to emerge. The brain acts like a processor, but one which relates whole concepts to one another and looks for similarities, differences, or relationships between them. It is not like a computer. It is much more powerful in that it does not assemble thoughts and feelings from bits of information in a true sense, but from sophisticated and intricate patterns. This new understanding of how the brain functions has challenged several longstanding assumptions about emotions. For example, psychologists once maintained that emotions were purely mental expressions generated by the brain alone. We now know that this is not true — emotions have as much to do with the body as they do with the brain. Single neurons in the brain alter their behaviour in response to the signals received from each heartbeat. In response, complexes of neurons in the brain change their grouping and firing patterns. They alter their behaviour in order to embed the information received from the heart and send it into the central nervous system. The information embedded within cardiac pulses alters central nervous function in behaviourally significant ways. There is, in fact, a two-way communication between heart and brain that shifts physiological functioning and behaviour in response to the information exchanged.

Furthermore, of the bodily organs, the heart plays a particularly important role in the emotional system. Analysis of information flow into the human body has shown that much of it impacts the heart **first**, flowing to the brain only after it has been perceived by the heart. It suggests our experience of the world at times is routed first through the heart, which 'thinks' about the experience and then sends the data to the brain for further processing — not the other way round. The heart routinely engages in what could be described as a 'neural conversation' with the brain and, in essence, the two act together in 'deciding' which actions to take. Emotions are thus a product of the brain, heart, and body acting as a team.

The science of neurocardiology has shown how the heart is a sensory organ and a sophisticated information encoding and processing centre, with an extensive intrinsic nervous system. Its circuitry enables it to learn, remember, and make functional decisions independent of the cranial brain. Moreover, numerous experiments have demonstrated that patterns of cardiac afferent neurological input to the brain not only affect physiological regulatory centres, but also influence higher brain centres involved in perception and emotional processing.

My interest for the last few years has been looking at heart–brain interactions through the measurement of heart rate variability analysis. Heart rate variability (HRV), derived from the electrocardiogram (ECG), is a measure of the naturally occurring beat-to-beat changes in heart rate. The analysis of HRV, or heart rhythms, provides a powerful, non-invasive measure of neurocardiac function. It can reflect heart–brain interactions and autonomic nervous system changes, which are particularly sensitive to changes in emotional states — providing a sort of 'picture' of an individual's internal emotional landscape. Findings from research suggest there is an important link between emotions and changes in the patterns of both efferent (descending) and afferent (ascending) autonomic nervous system (ANS) activity. These changes lead to dramatic changes in the pattern of the heart's rhythm, often without any change in the actual heart rate variability.

To give an example, during emotions such as anger, frustration, or anxiety, heart rhythms become more erratic and disordered, indicating less synchronisation in the ANS. In contrast, sustained positive emotions, such as appreciation, love, or compassion, are associated with highly ordered or coherent patterns in the heart rhythms, reflecting greater synchronisation between the ANS, and a shift in autonomic balance toward an increase in one aspect of that system known as parasympathetic activity (Figure 17.1).

In addition to understanding how complex ANS activity patterns correlate with differing emotions, there is now a better understanding of the role played by signals which flow from the heart and body to the brain and how they help generate and allow the experience of feelings and emotions. This was first noticed as far back as 1929 when it was found that stimulation

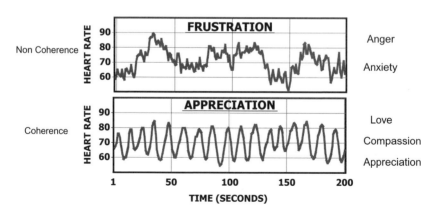

Figure 17.1   How perceptions and emotions affect autonomic nervous system balance and heart rhythm.

of a nerve connecting the heart to the brain — the vagus nerve — inhibited motor activity and prolonged sleep. Among the first modern psycho-physiological researchers to systematically examine the two-way dialogue between the heart and brain were John and Beatrice Lacey. During 20 years of research throughout the 1960s and 1970s, they observed that input from the heart and cardiovascular system could significantly affect perception and behaviour. Their research concluded that sensory–motor integration could be modified by cardiovascular activity. One interesting piece of research established relationships between the heart's signals to the brain and reaction times. For example, they showed that decreasing heart rate in the anticipatory period of reaction-time experiments quickened reaction times, while increasing heart rate slowed reaction times. They introduced the terms 'cortical facilitation' and 'cortical inhibition' to describe these effects. Since that time, experiments have demonstrated the role played by the heart in modulating many processes including pain perception, hormone production, and cognitive functions.

At that time, however, studies did not generally consider the role of emotion or how patterns of signals from the heart influenced emotional processes. Later, Professor Karl Pribram of Stanford University in the USA was the first to theorise that the brain functioned as a complex pattern identification and matching system. In his model, past experience builds within us a set of familiar patterns, which are maintained in our individual neural architecture. Inputs to the brain from both the external and internal environments contribute to the maintenance of these patterns. This includes the heart's rhythmic activity; digestive, respiratory and hormonal rhythms; and patterns of muscular tension, particularly facial expressions. These inputs are continuously monitored by the brain and help organise perception, feelings, and behaviour. According to his view, when an input pattern is sufficiently different from the familiar reference pattern, this 'mismatch' or departure from the familiar underpins the generation of feelings and emotions.

Monitoring the alterations in the rates, rhythms, and patterns of signals is thus a key function of the thinking and emotional systems in the brain. The heart, as a primary and consistent generator of rhythmic information patterns in the human body, and possessing a far more extensive communication system with the brain than other major organs, plays a particularly important role in this process. With each beat, the heart not only pumps blood, but also continually transmits dynamic patterns of neurological, hormonal, pressure, and electromagnetic information to the brain and throughout the body. These signals cascade up to a number of areas in the brain involved in the processing of emotion.

In particular, research supports the view that cardiac signals exert an important influence on central emotional processing. For example, they influence an area in the brain called the amygdala and its associated nuclei. These play an important role in storing and processing 'emotional' memory and in attaching emotional significance to sensory stimuli. Neural activity in the amygdala is synchronised to the cardiac cycle and is modulated by cardiovascular signals to that area in the brain via its neural connections.

Incoherent ('jagged') heart rhythm patterns produced by strong feelings of anxiety in an otherwise healthy individual contrast to coherent ('smooth') heart rhythm patterns. The latter are associated with positive emotions, and evoke feelings of security and wellbeing. This has led to the emergence of interventions capable of shifting the pattern of the heart's rhythmic activity in order to modify an individual's emotional state. These interventions have emerged in a number of different ways and with different labels, e.g. 'mindfulness', 'meditation', etc. The commonest of these is simply altering the breathing rhythm by taking several slow, deep breaths. Most individuals do not realise, however, the reason breathing techniques are effective in helping to shift one's emotional state is because changing one's breathing rhythm modulates the heart's rhythmic activity — it is a way of 'tricking' the heart into communicating a different signal to the emotional processing centres in the brain.

The modulation of the heart's rhythm by respiratory activity is referred to as respiratory sinus arrhythmia (RSA). Techniques researched and developed by an organisation in California in the USA, HeartMath® and its research wing, The Institute of HeartMath® under the research leadership of Dr Rollin McCraty, have for many years researched and employed heart-focussed interventions that also facilitate emotional shifts by generating changes in the heart's rhythmic patterns.

In this context, coherence is important in that different thoughts and different emotional states can be considered 'coherent' or 'incoherent'.

HeartMath® has demonstrated that positive emotions are associated with a higher degree of coherence with the heart's rhythmic activity. The term 'physiological coherence' has been used to describe a number of related physiological phenomena that are frequently associated with feelings of appreciation — i.e., positive emotion including a phenomenon referred to as 'resonance'.

In simple terms, when the human system is operating in the coherent mode, increased synchronisation occurs between nerves controlling automatic functions in the body (known as the autonomic nervous system), and a biological state known as entrainment occurs between the heart rhythms, respiration, and blood pressure is observed. This occurs because these biological subsystems all oscillate or vibrate, in a physiological sense, at the resonant frequency.

In humans and in many animals, the resonant frequency of this system is 0.1 hertz, which is equivalent to a 10-second rhythm. This resonance occurs when an individual is actively feeling appreciation or some other positive emotion, although resonance can also emerge during states of sleep and deep relaxation. In terms of physiological functioning, resonance confers a number of benefits to an individual's physiology. For example, there is increased cardiac output in conjunction with increased efficiency in fluid exchange, filtration, and absorption between the capillaries and tissues; increased ability of the cardiovascular system to adapt to circulatory requirements; and better communication between cells throughout the body. This results in increased physiological efficiency. These findings demonstrate a link between positive emotions and increased physiological efficiency, which may partly explain the growing number of correlations documented between positive emotions, improved health, and increased longevity.

How can an Individual Generate Physiological Coherence?

Although physiological coherence is a natural state that can occur spontaneously, sustained episodes are generally rare. While specific rhythmic breathing methods can induce coherence and associated entrainment for brief periods, cognitively-directed, paced breathing is difficult for most people to maintain. On the other hand, HeartMath® has found individuals can produce extended periods of physiological coherence by actively generating and sustaining a feeling of appreciation. Sincere feelings of appreciation appear to excite the system at its resonant frequency, allowing the coherent mode to emerge naturally. This typically makes it easier for people to sustain a positive emotion for much longer periods, thus facilitating the process of establishing and reinforcing coherent patterns as the familiar reference.

Once a new pattern is established, the brain strives to maintain a match with the new programme, thus increasing the probability of having an optimistic outlook and maintaining emotional stability, even during challenging situations, such as when an individual moves within or between the elements of the 4 cusps. Living with cancer carries many stresses, not least the follow up appointments at clinic. In addition, most people who have had a cancer diagnosis worry a lot when they develop new symptoms. HeartMath® have found that consciously generating feelings of love and appreciation while imagining you are 'breathing' through the area of the heart, for example, appears to confer a far wider range of benefits than simply 'forcing' coherence using breathing techniques alone.

During such states of coherence, bodily systems appear to function with a high degree of synchronisation, efficiency, and harmony and the body's natural regenerative processes appear to be facilitated. Psychologically, this mode is associated with improved cognitive performance, increased emotional stability, and enhanced psychosocial functioning and quality of life. Additionally, after practicing this mode for even short periods (days or weeks), many individuals report experiencing a notable reduction in inner mental dialogue and turmoil along with feelings of increased peace, self-security, and sustained positive emotion.

Researchers in a comparative study in the USA of survivors of breast cancer at Cusp A ('cured') measured participants' baseline heart-rate coherence (HRC) before the six-week study and final HRC after its completion. The study incorporated HeartMath® interventions to help individual generate coherence in HRV patterns. The results clearly showed a significant decrease in the amount of low HRC, which, of course, was an improvement; and significant increases in the amount of high HRC.

The researchers observed several themes during the study, firstly that the patients felt in control, secondly they were able to integrate processes into everyday life and lastly, what they termed 'emotional transformation' as evidenced in the women's subjective comments, e.g.:

- 'If nothing else, I am learning to control my emotions and that is having a tremendous impact on my life'.
- 'I know that happiness is a choice. I am going to try to track my feelings, thoughts, actions and start each day and end each day in a positive manner'.
- 'Remember when I used to cry a lot. I have noticed that I am not doing that now. I feel more centred'.
- 'You know, it is amazing in our society that we spend all this time and money on things, but we don't take the time to work on our greatest gifts: our heart and mind'.

Despite a small sample of women used for this study, the researchers said, the 'significant changes observed' would be clinically relevant if replicated in a larger sampling.

They said the almost immediate improvement in HRC levels using HeartMath's® interventions for establishing baseline HRC levels was very promising in managing stress and developing coping skills.

Managing Emotions with Cancer — The Difference between Positive 'Thinking' and Positive 'Feeling'

Although most people intuitively know they feel best and operate more efficiently and effectively when experiencing positive emotions, we do not generally and consistently engage such states in day-to-day living. This is especially the case when faced with a diagnosis of cancer and its associated treatments and/or palliative care. A main factor underlying this discrepancy is a fundamental lack of mental and emotional self-management skills. In other words, individuals generally do not make efforts to actively build greater emotional quality in their daily experiences because they simply 'don't know how'.

Various stress management practices have been developed to help individuals manage their emotions when facing illness, such as cancer. However, the majority of these approaches are based on a cognitive model in which all emotions follow a cognitive assessment of sensory input, leading to a behavioural response. Therefore, these approaches rely on strategies that engage or restructure cognitive processes. The basic theoretical framework is that if emotions always follow thought, then by changing one's thoughts, one can gain control over the emotions. However, research has made it clear that emotional processes operate at a much higher speed than thoughts, and frequently bypass the mind's reasoning process entirely. In other words, not all emotions follow thoughts; many (and in fact most in certain contexts) occur independently of the cognitive systems and can significantly influence the cognitive process and its output or feelings.

As a result, techniques that encourage **positive thinking** *without* also showing how to engage **positive feelings** frequently provide only temporary, if any, relief from emotional distress. While a conceptual shift may occur (which is important), the fundamental source of the emotional stress remains largely intact. This has significant implications for emotion regulation interventions and suggests that intervening at the level of the emotional system may in many cases be a more direct and efficient way to transform thoughts, feelings, and behaviours and instil more positive emotion.

HeartMath® developed techniques that aim to combine a shift in the focus of attention to the area around the heart (where many people subjectively feel positive emotions) with the intentional self-induction of a sincere positive emotional state, such as appreciation. They found appreciation is one of the most effective, powerful and easiest of the positive emotions for individuals to self-induce and sustain for longer periods. This shift in focus and feeling serves to increase heart rhythm coherence, which results in a change in the pattern of cardiac signals sent to the cognitive and emotional centres in the brain. This coupling of a more organised signal pattern with an intentionally self-generated feeling of appreciation reinforces the natural conditioned response between the physiological state and the positive emotion. Once this association is firmly conditioned, simply pretending to breathe through the area of the heart, during a challenging situation where it may be hard to 'pull positive thinking out of the air', can often facilitate an emotional shift. It requires training, practice and perseverance, but the affects can be dramatic.

Positive emotion-focused techniques can thus enable individuals to effectively replace stressful thought patterns and feelings with more positive perceptions and emotions when they are needed most. However, there are also benefits that extend beyond reducing stress and negative emotions in the present moment. Learning to self-generate positive emotions with increasing consistency can give rise to long-term improvements in emotion regulation abilities, attitudes, and relationships that affect many aspects of one's life. It may provide a means of regaining some control over situations that appear 'at the mercy' of drugs, physicians and disease.

It is believed these longer term benefits stem from the fact that, as individuals experience appreciation and its consequent physiological coherence with increasing consistency, the coherent patterns become ever more familiar to the brain. Thus, these patterns become established in the neural framework as a new, stable, baseline or norm which the system then strives to maintain. Therefore, when stress or emotional instability is subsequently experienced, the familiar coherent, stable state is more readily accessible, enabling a quicker and more enduring emotional shift. Through this blueprint process, positive emotions and coherent physiological patterns progressively replace maladaptive emotional patterns and stressful responses as the habitual way of 'being'.

The techniques I have outlined are intentionally designed as simple, easy-to-use interventions that can be adapted to virtually any culture or age group. They are independent of religious or cultural bias, and most individuals feel an enjoyable but emotional shift. It is possible to experience a broadened perception the first time of use. Most age groups can effectively use such techniques and there are organisations and tools for use in specific contexts available. These can be accessed in the further reading suggestions in this book.

Summary and Conclusion

The human body has an inherent capacity for self-healing and regeneration. However, life's hectic pace coupled with frequent inefficient mental and emotional activity can compromise the system's natural regenerative processes. The energy drains produced by unmanaged negative emotions influence and have an impact on our biological system, placing added stress on the entire body. This can contribute to conditions such as fatigue, burnout, and increased susceptibility to both infectious and chronic disease. The health implications are substantial, as there is now a large volume of evidence that the depletion of such emotional energy plays a major and largely unrecognised role in both the genesis and aggravation of many health problems.

By cultivating a state of psychophysiological coherence, positive emotion-focussed techniques help individuals create an internal environment that is conducive to both physical and emotional regeneration. There are numerous research studies providing support for this view, documenting both short-term and long-term health benefits associated with the use of positive emotion-focussed techniques.

Recent years have seen the emergence of a growing body of information linking positive emotions to the enhancement of human functioning and to the mind–body links involved in such functioning.

These findings substantiate what many individuals have intuitively known — that positive emotions not only feel good at the subjective level, but also bolster one's ability to meet life's challenges with grace and ease, and foster good health and wellbeing.

I have tried in this chapter to review how the brain functions as a complex pattern identification and matching system, and to highlight the role signals (particularly from the heart) play in establishing an individual's own, familiar, reference patterns. I have also shown that such patterns are critical in ultimately determining emotional experience.

Emotions are reflected in the heart's rhythm patterns and by initiating a change in heart rhythm patterns, it is possible to bring about rapid and significant changes in perception and our emotional experience. Positive emotion-focussed techniques that couple a change in the heart's rhythmic patterns by generating emotions such as appreciation have been shown to be an effective means of reducing stress and negative emotions and of instilling more positive perceptions, emotions, and behaviours. Furthermore, as individuals learn to sustain positive emotions and physiological coherence with consistent practice using tried and tested techniques, this results in increased physiological efficiency and emotional stability. While this will not, of course, change the diagnosis of cancer nor determine any prognosis it could provide an additional source of understanding and help by giving those embarking on this highly challenging emotional journey a means of influencing and managing those emotions.

If you decide this is a path you might wish to explore, the following further reading will allow you to access more information and methods of learning these techniques:

- Science of The Heart: Exploring the Role of the Heart in Human Performance, *An Overview of Research Conducted by the Institute of HeartMath* http://www.heartmath.org/research/science-of-the-heart/ introduction.html
- HeartMath UK http://heartmath.co.uk/
- HeartMath http://www.heartmath.com/about/company-information. html
- The HeartMath Solution http://www.heartmathstore.com/item/1064/ heartmath-the-heartmath-solution
- Emwave Coherence Monitor http://www.heartmathstore.com/item/ 6320/emwave2

Competing Interests

- Member of Scientific Board — Institute of HeartMath (IOHM)

Acknowledgements

- Rollin McCraty, Ph.D., Executive Vice President and Director of Research — IOHM
- Janet Tapsell — Cingulate Consulting Ltd

Chapter 18

Bereavement and Grief by the Rev. Gary Bradley and J R Smith

Bereavement is by definition the process we go through when we suffer loss of something or someone very special to us. In terms of this book, it therefore applies to the women diagnosed with cancer who are coping with the loss that this entails and to the relatives of the minority of women who will sadly succumb to their disease.

At the time of diagnosis, there is an enormous range of emotions at play. These range from denial, anger, grief, depression, aggression, numbness, etc. There is no doubting that at that first consultation, numbness and disbelief will be the strongest emotion, as well as 'why me'? 'I've done nothing to deserve this, I've eaten healthily, not smoked, not drank, it can't be true'. However, over the next few days/weeks when the management plan is clarified, there is the coping with loss of organs if surgery is planned; this may involve loss of fertility, or feelings of loss of womanhood and a true bereavement process unfolds. If this is the first major illness you have encountered, there will also be that loss of invincibility. I think we all feel invincible, thinking it will never happen to us, until it does — and that is a terrible shock. Anger may centre on 'why me? Why have I been dealt this hand of cards?' If you are religious, you may wonder why God has allowed this to happen to you.

Ironically, you may struggle most with the psychological sequelae of your disease at the end of the active treatment. Up until then, you and us, your carers, are completely focussed on the treatment in hand. At the end of treatment, when we are sitting in clinic, we tell the majority of patients that they are in complete remission. This is great news! We then tell you that you will come back to clinic in three months and every three months this year, four-monthly next year and six-monthly for the following three years. Then at that time, if all is well, you will be offered a choice of discharge or annual surveillance. This fits in with the 4 cusps and reaching 'the cured circle'.

However, let us return to this consultation at the end of treatment. You know on one level you should be happy, but you may well feel 'cast adrift'. We are patting you on the back saying 'it's all okay, off you go and live your life', when in fact a seismic shift has taken place in your whole life. This may well be when the emotional roller coaster starts!

This, therefore, tends to be the point where introduction of the grieving response most needs discussed. This response was first codified by Elizabeth Kubler-Ross, an American physician, into DABDA: D is for denial, A for anger, B for bewilderment, bargaining, D for depression, A for acceptance and H for hope (Figure 18.1). In her original work, there was no H; this was added later. Although Kubler-Ross did not suggest that these emotions were linear, i.e. occurring one after another, but that is very much how they came to be interpreted.

Things will never be the same again, but life can go on albeit differently.

A different model encompassing the same emotions is the 'tapestry of bereavement or a landscape of grief' (Figure 18.2). This model was developed by the Rev. Gary Bradley, co-author of this chapter and the Founder and chairman of the Westminster Bereavement Association.

The analogy here is with a picture. When you buy a picture, you will notice various features of that picture, and then as the picture hangs on

D	Denial
A	Anger
B	Bewilderment/bargaining
D	Depression
A	Acceptance
H	Hope

Figure 18.1   The grieving response.

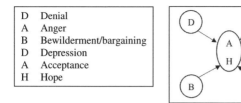

D	Denial
A	Anger
B	Bewilderment/bargaining
D	Depression
A	Acceptance
H	Hope

Figure 18.2   Sketch of the 'tapestry of bereavement/landscape of grief.

your wall, over time you notice different aspects of the picture until after some time you may hardly notice the picture at all, even although it is still there. You may, however, move the picture and it instantly becomes more visible.

The picture then is as shown in the sketch with the various emotions cropping up not in any particular order, but more randomly, with some predominating at one point and others at another. Over time, all of the parts of the tapestry fade and while they do not disappear, the tapestry becomes your new reality. This is when you have arrived at 'acceptance' and 'hope'.

This may all appear somewhat negative, but one of the amazing and heartening things many people say to me is that their cancer diagnosis finally gave them great inner strength and that they went on to do things that they know they would not otherwise have done. This is the concept of winning through losing — a very difficult place to get to, but something that can be genuinely empowering for the individual.

For those who lose a spouse, relative or close friend, the same range of emotions will occur and the tapestry is similar. The 'tapestry' by its flexibility and its ability to fade and then come back into focus may be a useful model for you to think around.

There is one further pictorial model of the grieving process (Figure 18.3), which you may find useful, particularly if you have got stuck in a bad place. This model has been developed by Dr Nicola Holtom, a Palliative Care specialist in Norwich. She kindly gave permission for it to be used.

If you get stuck at the bottom of the loop, you can get out, even although when you are there, you may not believe it. As you now know, much of this book is about strategies to get out to the sunlit uplands of acceptance and hope.

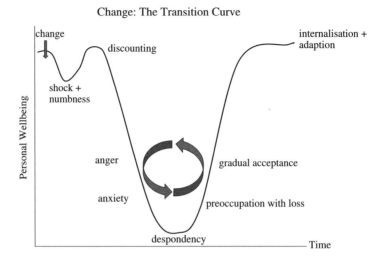

Figure 18.3   The grieving process, by Dr Nicola Holtom.

This process, particularly when one arrives at hope and acceptance, ties in with the next Venn diagram of psychology, spirituality and religion in Chapter 19 (Figure 19.2). Psychology, spirituality and religion are the areas that most will choose to explore further.

Chapter 19

Spiritual Approaches to Living with Cancer by J R Smith

You may consider it brave, foolhardy, presumptuous or just plain not appropriate for a doctor such as me to even enter into this subject. My reason for including a chapter on this subject is that over the last two plus decades I have had the privilege to look after a large number of women who have either been cured of their cancer or have lived with their cancer for a long time before succumbing to the disease. I have become quite convinced that religion and spirituality allows people to cope better with their disease than those who see things in strictly secular, non-religious terms. The term spirituality is used, as meaning, the attempt to experience a sense of the transcendental, independent of religion. I would not dream of suggesting that I think that those with religion live longer with their disease, but I do believe that particularly for those who are living with cancer many of them do 'live better'. You may think when you start this chapter that 'I'm somebody who's not religious or spiritual so there's no point in reading this', or that you are religious and once again, therefore, there's not much point in reading it because how does one change the way that one is? I think it is also important that I state here at the start of this chapter that I have no agenda whatsoever to proselytize for any specific religion. I myself could have been regarded as a non-practicing Christian for the first 35 years of my life and since then have practiced, or at least tried to, Christianity in a liberal Anglo-Catholic tradition. I do also have a keen interest in Eastern Orthodoxy, in particular in aspects concerned with Christian mysticism. I impart this information not through any desire to suggest that what I do is better than what anybody else does, but merely to be clear to you in my own position. Ironically, it has been the juxtaposition of looking after patients with cancer and HIV, watching their coping mechanisms and having to develop some of my own, coupled with a brief but severe bout of personal illness, and difficulty which propelled me along my own personal route.

One of the things which I have been struck by is the common ground between the major religions: Christianity, Judaism, Islam, Hinduism and Buddhism. Mandalas, for example, are found in many of these religions (see Figure 19.1). To my mind, in health terms, the type of religious belief

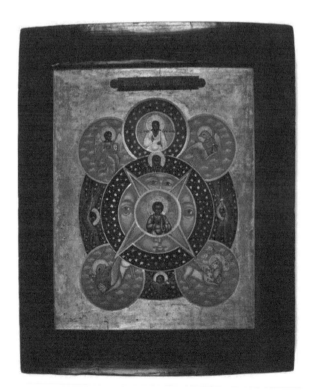

Figure 19.1   Picture of a Christian mandala: the all seeing eye of God.

is unimportant. What does matter is the belief itself. Apart from the moral code, one of the unifying themes of all religions is that they all have a monastic element, and for that small group of 'holy people', be they men or women, there is a unifying feature of 'seeking the light'. Until I read around this area, I had never realised that the common saying to 'see the light' was a reference to that other-worldly light. The Greek and Russian hesychast monk enters via asceticism and repetitive prayer into a trance like state to see the light. Renaissance art obsesses with 'the light', the white dove, the Holy Spirit of the Trinity. The Soufi Moslem seeks the light as does the Buddhist yogi. This light is that which is sought by the holy of all religions. That holy is spelt with an 'H', but, it could just as easily be spelt with a 'Wh', wholly. I cannot believe that all these holy people, whatever their tradition, are seeing different 'lights'.

Surely, it can be no coincidence that many of those patients who have had near death-experiences describe seeing a light and that they felt as if they were going on a journey into the light.

I have had patients from all of these belief systems and there is undoubtedly a common thread running through all of the world's major religions. When it comes to living with cancer, they all seem to have the capacity to provide reassurance and hope in equal measure to each other. It is noteworthy that hospitals historically, certainly in the Western tradition, grew out of monasteries where there was a belief in tending to the physical, emotional and religious wellbeing of those being cared for. To my mind, this is one of the failings of modern medicine, that as we have got far better at achieving higher cure rates, and have much more to offer as every year goes by, we have left the care of the spiritual side of the patient behind as a matter of almost irrelevance. Worse than this, it is almost impossible to enter the arena of religion with your patient without a serious danger of being seen as a proselytiser, something which I have absolutely no intention or desire to be seen as.

I have been interested for many years in the work of Carl Gustav Jung, the famous Swiss psychologist. I do think that Jung saw the link between psychology and religion and his insights came partly through dream analysis. Jung coined the term 'individuation', by which he meant that process by which a person becomes a psychological individual, that is a separate, indivisible unity or 'whole' meaning that the person has come to selfhood or self-realisation. He firmly believed that people only got to this place and became in psychoanalytical terms 'mature' when for most individuals they passed the age of 40. Jung's view on dreams is much more interesting than any dictionary definition: 'The dream is the little hidden door in the innermost and most secret recesses of the psyche,… All consciousness separates; but in dreams we put on the likeness of that more universal, truer, more eternal man dwelling in the darkness of primordial night'. Jung believed in the collective subconscious. The subconscious is that place that can be entered by achieving a dreamlike or trance like state. Many religious ceremonies achieve this with the combination of ritual, chanting, a mixture of sights, sounds and smells, which have the capacity to induce a semi-hypnotic state. The current obsession with yoga is almost certainly tapping into something similar. Chapters 14 and 15 in this book deal with hypnotherapy, meditation etc.

I always find it interesting that when you read works by religious authors they always feel that any reference to psychotherapy or hypnotherapy as having aspects bearing on religion is somehow an insult to that religion. Conversely, the psychologist wishes to avoid entering the arena of religion. It is the forbidden zone. I have never really understood why entering into the subconscious, be it via a hypnotherapy session, seeing a psychologist or partaking in a religious ceremony that allows one access to your god, should be seen in anything other than positive terms.

It is noteworthy that when Jung was questioned in public about whether he believed in God himself he replied, "I do not believe in God.…" and then paused. After what seemed an age he continued, "I know".

In addition to the mainstream religions there are also individuals who are spiritual healers who may come from shamanistic or pagan belief systems or utilise aspects of Buddhism or aspects of Christianity. I personally refer those patients who are interested in a spiritual approach and who have no religion to a spiritual healer who combines some aspects of the Buddhist and Christian traditions; he has often worked wonders. For those who are lapsed from their original religion they may wish to revisit it. For those who are less interested in these aspects, then the help of counsellors or psychologists to find the inner self and inner peace again can be helpful.

The great difficulty is how to get into the subject in the first place with your patients and this is something, by my own experience, which is only

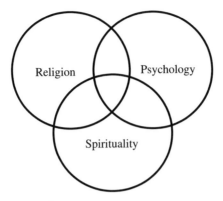

Figure 19.2   Crossover between spirituality, psychology and religion.

sometimes possible and almost always when I have truly got to know the patient. Even then, entering the discussion can be fraught with difficulty, again relating back to the danger of being seen as a proselytiser. The irony is that if one finds that somebody has no religion, then the route is certainly not to suggest that they start going to church or going to their local temple, but rather that they go down the psychological route. The enormous success of Deepak Chopra's books, *Mind Body Healing* etc. are ample testimony to the unmet need here.

Figure 19.2 uses a Venn diagram to show the crossover between spirituality, psychology and religion, demonstrating separateness as well as the crossover. I regularly use this diagram to enter the subject with patients without causing offence. Some time ago I pushed this drawing over the table during a consultation to a young women who had recently had a hysterectomy for cancer. I said to her "Do any of these things appeal to you?" She looked at the Venn diagram, smiled and said "My brother is a priest and I'm right into religion, I'm a pretty spiritual person and as of last week I've signed up with a psychotherapist". I laughed, she laughed and we both agreed she had it well taped!

I have written a book *The Journey: A Pathway to Spiritual Fulfilment* (in press) which explores many of these issues further. I have also put some suggested further reading on page 228 for those who wish to explore this area further!

Chapter 20

Conclusion

It may seem strange to finish a book such as this with some conclusions. However, the book started with some key aims:

1. Most important to me is that you have gained accurate information. This, ironically, is not easy in our current situation of masses of information, but much of it highly dubious.

2. When you are told you have cancer, you (along with everybody else) will have thought, 'I'm going to die very soon'. This is virtually never the case — the vast majority of people are in Cusps A and B, i.e. 'cured' or 'living with cancer' NOT preterminal (Cusp C) or dying (Cusp D).

3. All of you will experience grief/bereavement after diagnosis, although most of you will live for long periods of time after this and the majority will be cured. The landscape of grief may prove to be a useful model for you to remember during your darker moments. What you are experiencing is normal.

4. That you can see the different strands of orthodox medicine and complementary medicine and how in each of these spheres some things will be right for you and others not, but that you, in conjunction with your doctors, nurses and therapists will find what is right for you in the knowledge that you know what is available.

5. That if you are of a religious/spiritual frame of mind, you persevere with this, expand it and if you are not you either go down the route of psychological intervention (either by the orthodox route of clinical

psychology or the complimentary route e.g. hypnotherapy) or if this is not your way, utilise practical approaches (e.g. cardiac sychronicity). The three patients who wrote pieces typify, by pure chance on my part, these different approaches.

6. The diagnosis of cancer changes your life and that of your family and close friends forever, but to quote Maggie Keswick Jencks again 'Above all, what matters is not to lose the joy of living in the fear of dying'.

Chapter 21

Suggested Further Reading

Websites have been suggested throughout the book and you may find Ovarian Cancer Action, McMillan and Marie Curie valuable resources.

Useful Addresses

www.adjuvantsite.com
(program for estimation of risk and benefits of adjuvant therapy)

www.minervation.com/cancer/breast/professional/
(UK National Electronic Library for Health information on breast cancer)

CancerBACUP

3, Bath Place
Rivington Street
London, EC2A 3JR
Tel: 0808 800 1234
http://www.cancerbacup.org.uk/

Cancer Research UK
PO Box 123
Lincoln's Inn Fields
London, WC2A 3PX
Tel: 020 7242 0200
Fax: 02 07269 3100
www.cancerresearchuk.org/aboutcancer/specificcancers/93645
www.crc.org.uk/cancer/Aboutcan_common2.html

The following books are slightly more eclectic!

1. Lawrence van der Post, *Jung and the story of our time.* Vintage 2002.
2. C G Jung, *The Undiscovered Self.* Routledge 1996.
3. *The Way of a Pilgrim* translated and annotated Glebb Pocrowsky. Dart and Longman Todd 2001.
4. C G Jung, *Memories, Dream, Reflections.* Fontana Press 1995.
5. C G Jung, *Modern Man in Search of a Soul.* Routledge *2001.*
6. Jennifer Lash, *On pilgrimage.* Bloomsbury 1998.
7. Arnold Mindel, *The Shaman's Body.* Harper San Francisco 1993.
8. Thomas Merton, *The Intimate Merton.* Lion 2002.
9. Sogyal Rinpoche, *The Tibetan Book of Living and Dying.* Random House 1992.
10. Deepak Chopra, *Quantum Healing. Bantam* 1989.
11. Bernie Siegel, *Love, Medicine and Miracles.* Arrow 1988.
12. Laurens Van Der Post, *The Seed and the Sower.* Hogarth Press 1963.
13. John Diamond. *Snake Dance.*
14. Cassandra Marks, *Homeopathy: A Step by Step Guide.* Element Books 1997.
14. Michael Geerin-Tosh, *Living proof, a medical mutiny.* Scribner 2002.
15. www.jrsmithgynaecology.com: this provides a comprehensive description of all the operations described in this book with art work by Dee MacLean.
16. Viktor Frankl. *Man's Search For Meaning* Ebury Press, Random House, London 1959, 2004.
17. www.viktorfrankl.org
18. J Richard Smith. *The Journey: A Pathway to Spiritual Fulfilment* (in press 2016).

Glossary

Appendix: 'Worm-like' structure in the bowel

Cervix: Neck of the womb

CIN: Cervical intraepithelial neoplasia

-ectomy: Removal of an organ (e.g. appendicectomy)

Endometrium: Lining of the womb

Fallopian tube: The 'tube' between the uterus and ovary

FIGO: Federation International Gynaecologie Oncologie; an international committee which advises on 'staging' of diseases — see *parametrium stage* below

HPV: Human papilloma virus

Lymph nodes: Glands that are situated alongside blood vessels

Metastasis (plural = metastases): Cancer that has spread from its primary (original) site, also known as secondary cancer

Omentum: Fatty structure hanging from the large bowel

-ostomy: to fashion a hole in an organ (e.g. colostomy: to fashion a hole in the colon (large bowel))

Ovaries: The organs that produce eggs. When they stop working is when the menopause arrives

Parametrium stage: The amount which a cancer has spread; always I, II, III or IV, I being the earliest (i.e. not spread) and IV the latest (i.e. spread widely)

Primary cancer: The place from where the cancer has started

Secondary cancer: Cancer that has spread from its original, primary site; also known as metastases

SIL: Squamous intra-epithelial lesion, the American equivalent word for CIN

Uterus: Womb

VAIN: Vaginal intra-epithelial neoplasia; a pre-cancerous condition of the vaginal skin

VIN: Vulval intra-epithelial neoplasia; a pre-cancerous condition of the vulva

Vulva: The skin on the outside of the vagina, encompassing the labia Majora (hair bearing skin), the labia minora (the inner lips) and the clitoris

Index

Cut-out 4 cusp diagram

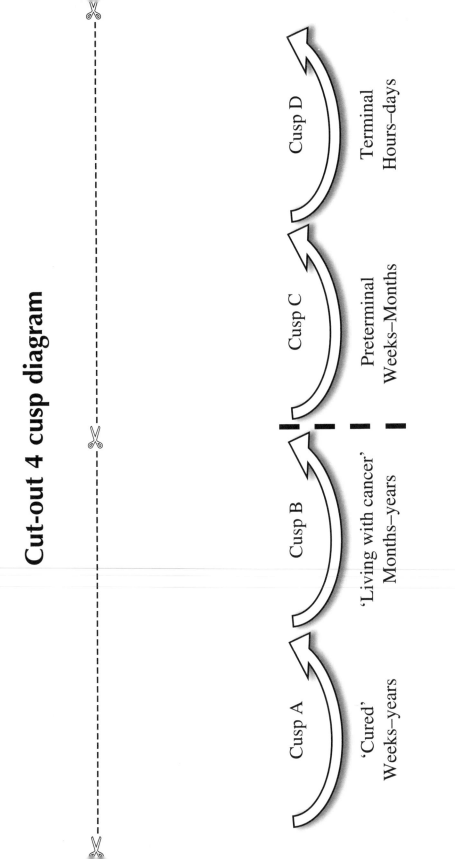

Cusp A
'Cured'
Weeks–years

Cusp B
'Living with cancer'
Months–years

Cusp C
Preterminal
Weeks–Months

Cusp D
Terminal
Hours–days